Pain

Pain

A handbook for nurses

Second edition

Beatrice Sofaer
Reader in Nursing
Brighton Polytechnic

CHAPMAN & HALL
London · Glasgow · New York · Tokyo · Melbourne · Madras

Published by Chapman & Hall, 2–6 Boundary Row, London SE1 8HN

Chapman & Hall, 2–6 Boundary Row, London SE1 8HN, UK

Blackie Academic & Professional, Wester Cleddens Road, Bishopbriggs, Glasgow G64 2NZ, UK

Chapman & Hall, 29 West 35th Street, New York NY10001, USA

Chapman & Hall Japan, Thomson Publishing Japan, Hirakawacho Nemoto Building, 7F, 1–7–11 Hirakawa-cho, Chiyoda-ku, Tokyo 102, Japan

Chapman & Hall Australia, Thomson Nelson Australia, 102 Dodds Street, South Melbourne, Victoria 3205, Australia

Chapman & Hall India, R. Seshadri, 32 Second Main Road, CIT East, Madras 600 035, India

First edition 1984
Second edition 1992

© 1984, 1992 Beatrice Sofaer

Typeset in 10/12 Plantin by Columns of Reading Ltd.
Printed in Great Britain by Page Bros (Norwich) Ltd.
ISBN 0 412 44010 5

A catalogue record for this book is available from the British Library

Library of Congress Cataloging-in-Publication data available

For Annie T. Altschul and the Sofaer family,
who all supported three years 'of pain' during a
study about pain.

'Pain is'
(Wall, 1977)

Wall, P. D. (1977) Why do we not understand pain?, in *The Encyclopaedia of Ignorance* (eds R. Duncan and M. Weston-Smith) Pergamon Press, pp. 361–368

Contents

Preface

The first edition of this book was written in Jerusalem in 1984. At that time I made an analogy between the old and the new in that beautiful city, and of how little and how much man has progressed in life and in 'pain relief'. It can be said, I think, that in general there has been an increased awareness in the nursing profession, and some progress in education has been made, towards an understanding of pain and its relief since the first edition of this book. But there is still much work to be done, and we can not afford to be complacent. Many people still suffer unnecessary pain.

As with the previous edition, this book is an attempt to introduce nurses to the concept of pain. Because nurses more than any other members of the health care team encounter pain in so many situations, it is of particular importance that we improve our knowledge. The medical profession is also taking note of the need for pain management with patients, and also the pressing need for education of nurses and doctors. (Report of The Royal College of Surgeons of England and The College of Anaesthetists, 1990). The International Association for the Study of Pain (1991) has just published its first suggestions for a core curriculum for professional education in pain.

The management of pain may prove difficult due to its subjective nature and because there are many factors influencing its expression and relief. Even though several disciplines have undertaken research into the nature of pain, its complexity still presents a challenge. In recent years there has been an acknowledgement that patients need to have their pain understood in a wide context. This understanding includes knowledge of physiology, the psychological and cultural factors which may influence pain, assessment techniques, and therapies. The content of this book is intended to introduce the reader to those topics. It is concerned more with general principles of pain management than with 'special types' of pain related to particular conditions or illnesses.

I have tried to make the text appealing to all grades of staff, and have attempted to avoid complicated jargon, as well as to bridge the gap between principles of awareness of patients' pain by nurses and some of the therapies. I debated with myself and colleagues about the wisdom of leaving in the interview in Chapter 1, but I was persuaded to leave it in by a colleague who reviewed the book and commented that it 'ought to be compulsory reading for all nurses'. I have, however, supported some of the examples in the case-study by material which is discussed later in the book.

References have been updated, and a general bibliography and reading list are provided at the end of the book.

An attempt has been made to include some simple explanations regarding the neurophysiological aspects of pain. Readers who have a particular interest may wish to follow up the references quoted. I feel it is of greater importance that nurses, for whom this book is primarily intended, are encouraged to be more aware of factors that fall within the realms of psychology and interpersonal communication. Nurses deal with ill people who are undergoing stressful periods in their lives. Since we are in a position to provide relief to patients, it follows that we should be aware of ways to assess pain with patients, and to know what options are available for relief. One option, for example, may be communicating with a medical colleague in order that a medication might be prescribed or changed to an alternative, while another might be to implement a non-invasive therapy. Whatever the option (or options), the nurse must have the necessary background knowledge and confidence so that the patient will not experience unnecessary suffering. As Melzack (1988) has stated, 'Pain can have a major impact on morbidity and mortality, it can mean the difference between life and death.'

My thanks to my family and colleagues, who have offered me encouragement. I am particularly grateful to Dr Janet Walker, Ms Hazel Platzer, and Dr John Lamberty for reading the first edition and discussing changes with me. I appreciate the thoughts and ideas shared by Dr John Carey and Dr Andrew Polmear, particularly for their helpful suggestions on the chapter on therapies. Finally, my grateful thanks to my colleague Professor Roger Morgan for help with proof-reading.

I hope you will find this introductory book helpful, and that you will feel encouraged to seek further information and knowledge.

Beatrice Sofaer
Brighton 1992

References

International Association for the Study of Pain (1991) Fields, H. L. (ed.), Core curriculum for professional education in pain. IASP Publications, Seattle.

Melzack, R. (1988) The tragedy of needless pain: a call for social action, in *Proc. 5th World Congress on Pain* (eds R. Dubner, G. F. Gebhart and M. R. Bond), Elsevier, Amsterdam, pp. 1–11.

Report of the Working Party on Pain after Surgery (1990) Royal College of Surgeons of England and College of Anaesthetists, London.

1

A patient's experience

I now equate hospitals with *pain*, really, and before I thought they were fairly pleasant places and that they [the staff] were there to look after you. I must admit I have a different opinion now, totally.

(A patient – 2½ weeks following surgery)

During a research project to assess the effect of an educational programme for nurses on postoperative pain of patients (Sofaer, 1985), which led to the first edition of this book, time was made available for staff on four surgical wards to listen to and comment on the experience of a patient who had undergone surgery. Several nurses felt uncomfortable and/or embarrassed on behalf of their profession while listening to the tape, but most agreed that this patient's experience was by no means exceptional.

A transcript of the interview is reproduced below exactly as it occurred. The woman was aged 38, married, and with three children. She was a civil servant by profession.

Some readers may feel that a single interview cannot be taken as representative of all patients' hospital experiences. However, one bad experience in this day and age is one too many. Many of the points discussed later in the book are highlighted by this experience.

Interview

Interviewer Thank you very much for letting me come to see you. I understand that you have been in hospital recently.

Respondent Yes, I was admitted for an operation because of a duodenal ulcer which I had for ten years. It had given no problems but, because of a new medication, the operation suddenly became necessary and I was admitted to hospital three weeks ago.

Interviewer	So you had your operation how long ago?
Respondent	On the 16th of November.
Interviewer	That's about what, about 16 days ago?
Respondent	That'll be it.
Interviewer	And, generally speaking, what were the main problems you experienced in hospital? For example, did you have any difficulty in sleeping at all?
Respondent	After the first night I had constant difficulty in sleeping. The medication provided in my case didn't seem to work and I could find no comfortable position and, since the pain-killers didn't work, nights were more or less spent sitting up in bed, changing to an armchair and generally wandering around the ward. The nurses (students) were very helpful but were, in most cases, unable to do anything since they had no authority to provide any alternative medication from that prescribed.
Interviewer	Did they report it to the trained staff?
Respondent	They said they had and when I actually spoke to the doctors they said yes, they were prescribing a different medication but, for some reason or other, it was never forthcoming at the appropriate time because my main problem obviously was that during the day it's much easier to put up with things simply because you can change position, you can move, you don't feel so hemmed in by your bed.
Interviewer	So you didn't get much sleep?
Respondent	No, very little.
Interviewer	How many days before your operation were you admitted?
Respondent	I was admitted one day before. I found the whole day a total waste of time because I went in at 10 o'clock in the morning and nothing was done until 5 o'clock in the evening.
Interviewer	Did anyone tell you what was going to happen to you at the operation?
Respondent	No, had I not consulted my own doctor about the operation, I would never have been aware of what it entailed. When I had gone originally to the hospital, they had simply said an operation for duodenal ulcer. I assumed it was being removed. It was my own doctor who explained that they were simply cutting the nerves which control the acidity in the stomach, otherwise I would never have known. On the evening before the operation a doctor

did explain at that point, when I was already in hospital, what was being done but he gave no indication of how I would feel afterwards. I assumed I would have the operation, perhaps feel a bit sore for a couple of days and then all would be past. I was not prepared for the amount of pain that there would be afterwards, definitely not, and I would have liked to be prepared for that.

Interviewer Did the nurses explain what would happen to you when you went to theatre?

Respondent The anaesthetist did. That's one thing I must admit, the anaesthetist was very, very kind. He explained everything. He came and visited every day afterwards for about four or five days and explained very clearly exactly what was going to be done in the way of anaesthetics, so on that score I must admit he was very, very conscientious.

Interviewer But what about the nursing staff, did you have any information at all from them?

Respondent No, they took it very much for granted, perhaps because I wasn't nervous at all. I had no idea what it entailed and therefore wasn't nervous. Perhaps had I been more nervous they would have spent time explaining or calming me, but I really didn't feel I needed any.

Interviewer You say you weren't nervous. If I said to you, 'Imagine a scale from 1 to 20, with 1 being not at all anxious, and 20 being extremely anxious before the operation', what score would you give youself?

Respondent Oh, I don't think more than six or seven, definitely. I was more upset at the fact of being away from my children for a week. The actual thought of the operation did not bother me at all.

Interviewer How long were you in for altogether?

Respondent From Sunday to Saturday, six days in all.

Interviewer Had you been in hospital before?

Respondent Only for pregnancies, I thoroughly enjoyed that.

Interviewer Have you ever had any painful experiences?

Respondent No, simply childbirth.

Interviewer How would you rate this last experience postoperatively, very painful, moderately painful, or a little pain . . .?

Respondent Extremely painful. I had no idea I could have taken so much pain for such a length of time, I really hadn't. I didn't realize. Quite frankly I couldn't believe it was happening at the time. I felt it had to stop at some point, there was so much discomfort. Not discomfort, that's the wrong word, pain. I can't say discomfort because it was very, very painful. The pain-killers I was getting didn't seem to work. I don't know why but they didn't, they worked for everyone else.

Interviewer   Had you been anxious about having pain before?

Respondent   It never entered my head that I would suffer pain in the hospital. I assumed that sedation was so effective nowadays, it had never occurred to me that I would feel anything beyond twinges or slight aches, certainly not the throbbing and incessant pain that I had. It was 24 hours really.

Interviewer   And the pain relief that you got, was that better than you expected, about what you expected, or less than you expected?

Respondent   Oh, far less than expected. After the first 24 hours you are expected to sit up and put up with everything. I felt I was expected to. The pain relief that was available was not effective for me. They were willing to give tablets but they were no good to me. In fact, I think I felt worse. Everyone else seemed to find they worked. For me they certainly didn't.

Interviewer   Did you mention it at all to the nursing staff?

Respondent   Yes, I didn't have much of a voice after the operation but I did do my best to mention it to the nursing staff and in each case they said that this was what was prescribed, that the tablets were equally effective compared to the injection or whatever it was I had been given before, and that the injection was too addictive. I wouldn't be allowed injections any more and this was the only alternative.

Interviewer   How many injections did you have, do you remember?

Respondent   That I can remember. One that I am aware of, because I had been fighting rather groggily with night staff at that point. It must have been the night after the operation. I remember trying to argue that I was in pain and I would like something. I remember them telling me it wasn't time, I couldn't have anything, and offering me two tablets and, I don't know why, I must have got it into my head that I had to have this injection at that point. I remember that very vaguely.

Interviewer   This was the night of your operation?

Respondent   The night yes, following the day when I had the operation.

I must have been given some kind of sedation during the day but that I don't remember. I seem to remember opening my eyes at various points. The pain really started during the night after the operation.

Interviewer   And are you telling me that the night staff refused to give you medication?

Respondent   They said it *wasn't time*. I would be able to have something later. Eventually, they said, 'Right, we are going to give you an injection now', and I remember being turned over, given an injection and next thing I remember it was morning. But after that there were no more injections, I was simply offered two tablets.

Interviewer   This was the day after your operation?

Respondent   Yes, yes.

Interviewer   And these were ineffective?

Respondent   Oh yes, I tested them myself. I didn't know whether I was just being difficult, so when they removed the various tubes and I did feel slightly better but was offered a pain-killer, I took them to see how I felt and I felt worse. I obviously couldn't tolerate these pain-killers for some reason. I tried to explain this but nobody seemed to believe it. They seemed to work for everyone else and so they *ought* to have worked for me, but they didn't, they definitely didn't. I wasn't imagining it.

Interviewer   So you are saying in fact that the nursing staff didn't believe you.

Respondent   Yes. They didn't seem to believe that this could possibly happen. I caught the doctor at one point. I was utterly desperate and croaked to him because I couldn't speak properly, but I tried to make myself understood. I said that I had tried taking the tablets but they didn't work. I was having too much pain to put up with, could he *please* prescribe something that would help and he said, 'Oh, in that case we'll prescribe injections'. Well, when night time came, and round came the medicine trolley, no injection had been prescribed and I was offered the same two tablets which I refused because they made me feel worse; and that was it really. It was a battle until more or less the last day when I had begun to feel that I could do without something. I just wanted to get home and try to take paracetamol or Disprin or something that would act as a

	pain-killer and, in fact, I think I got more relief with Disprin than I did with the famous two tablets.
Interviewer	Did you mention this at all to the trained staff – to the nursing sister or the staff nurse?
Respondent	Sisters I found were totally unsympathetic. The student nurses at least were ready to listen and, in fact, in cases agreed because I heard two say, 'You know, it's a shame when sedation has been prescribed, I don't see why it can't be given'. I remember that quite clearly at one point. Sisters, they had absolutely no idea of sitting down and listening – you would do this and you would do that and the pills must work – and no, absolutely no sympathy of any sort. They were very brisk. They seemed to see everything as a sick person's fantasy. I don't know – I found I got a lot more sympathy from the students, a lot more understanding from the students. They seemed to be able to relate better to your position than the sisters did. It was quite an eye-opener really, I now equate hospitals with *pain*, really, and before I thought they were fairly pleasant places, that they [the staff] were there to look after you. I must admit I have a different opinion now, totally.
Interviewer	Nobody discussed pain with you before the operation?
Respondent	No, no, no, no.
Interviewer	Would you have liked someone to?
Respondent	Oh, I think so, yes, because I don't think I am particularly intolerant to pain and I am sure I can put up with it as well as the next person. It's just the fact that it was so unexpected and it lasted for so long.
Interviewer	And so unrelieved?
Respondent	Yes, unrelieved, you almost felt like smashing your fist into something, simply to relieve the frustration of having to put up with this and not being able to get any help. I simply felt as if it was a nightmare and eventually I was going to have to waken up and find myself somewhere else. I remember thinking that quite clearly at one point.
Interviewer	When did you get out of bed, do you remember?
Respondent	The day after the operation, yes.
Interviewer	And were you offered any medicine before you got out?
Respondent	No, no. Pain-killers came only at particular times – at about two o'clock in the afternoon and then at night when the night staff came on. They were *very* fixed times, there was nothing in between.

Interviewer	You had pain in between the drug trolley rounds?
Respondent	Yes.
Interviewer	Did you ask for pain relief?
Respondent	I asked once after something had been done to the tubes in my stomach which brought on extra pain. I was more or less paralysed. I was finding it very difficult to walk and was told I would have to walk up and down, so I said, 'Could I have something to help?' and I got those two tablets after a lot of discussion with the sister on duty at the time. She said that moving the tubes shouldn't have caused any extra pain at all. It hadn't on one but it had on the other. I was having an awful lot of pain on one side which made it very difficult to move one leg and after a lot of discussion she seemed to go away and unlock something.
Interviewer	Was the discussion with you or with the staff?
Respondent	With me, with me.
Interviewer	And how did you find her manner on that occasion?
Respondent	Unsympathetic. This was *not* the time to take pain-killers. Pain-killers were given at certain times. I *certainly* shouldn't have any need of them at this point in the day.
Interviewer	This is what she said to you?
Respondent	Yes, yes. And I said, 'If I have to walk and I have been told that I have to walk, I can't walk unless I get something to help me ease the pain down one side, because since you have adjusted the tubes my left side is very much more painful and I find it difficult to move'. Eventually she did go and get something.
Interviewer	Generally speaking, do you think that nurses care a lot about pain relief, they care adequately about pain relief, or they could care more about pain relief?
Respondent	Nurses?
Interviewer	I mean generally, as a group.
Respondent	As a group? I don't think it comes very high on the list of priorities, no. It didn't seem to. There's a lot of care taken in washing and changing beds and keeping things clean. But no, pain didn't seem to be considered at all really. No one ever said, 'Are you in much discomfort, are you having any trouble?' – not really. There were exceptions, obviously, but on the whole, I'd have to say no.
Interviewer	Was there anything that you can remember that *was*

	helpful in relieving the pain the first few days after the operation?
Respondent	No. Simply the injections which had been given immediately after the operation seemed to be the only thing that really worked and there was only one that I remember being given. No, nothing seemed to work. Oh, another thing. I wish I had been told that I would suffer so much with wind after. I had no idea. I couldn't understand what these awful pains were creeping up my back until one of the other patients told me, 'Oh, this is normal, you get wind after you've had an operation, it's very painful and you have to break wind in some way or other'. I'd like to have known about that because no one thought to tell me I was having wind pain as well as, I presume, the usual aches and pains you have after an operation and I couldn't understand what this was. It was left to other patients who had already had operations and they said, 'Oh, these are wind pains and if you try walking and bending and taking drinks of hot water it ought to help to relieve the discomfort'. I would like to have been told that before. I'd have known what to expect.
Interviewer	Was it difficult for you to talk to the staff at all? Did you feel at ease asking questions of the nursing staff?
Respondent	After I had been in about four or five days, yes. I was more or less comfortable when it was time to go home.
Interviewer	When it was time to go home?
Respondent	When it was time to go home I felt I could talk to people because, I think it's the same anywhere, when we see a familiar face we tend to open up a bit more. At first, no, no, there was nobody I could really speak to. Because of losing my voice, I was at a disadvantage as well because I didn't feel like speaking.
Interviewer	How did you indicate to the staff that you were in pain then? Did you screw your face up?
Respondent	Oh, no, I could speak. I could whisper and they could hear but it was an effort talking and obviously I couldn't perhaps fight for things the way I might have if I had more of a voice and had it been less of an effort to speak.
Interviewer	You remember earlier on when we were chatting, I asked you to choose a score between 1 and 20, 1 being not very anxious and 20 being extremely anxious?
Respondent	Yes.

Interviewer	Bearing in mind this recent experience, if you had to go into hospital again for a similar sort of operation, what score would you give yourself?
Respondent	Assuming I went in the first place, it would be 20 definitely. I think I now have a *fear* of hospitals which I certainly did *not* have in the first place. On previous occasions I found hospitals very happy and pleasant places to be in, really. No, I really would be very unsure of ever going in again unless everything is explained and I know *exactly* what's going to happen first and have been assured that afterwards there will be the minimum discomfort possible, but I certainly would not go in very readily. It would have to be more or less a question of life and death I think.
Interviewer	You sound as if you had a pretty bad time.
Respondent	I didn't *believe* it. I didn't *believe* it was happening when it was happening. I really would have to talk to other people and find out if they felt the same way. I don't think they did. The other patients, they seemed to find, most of them, the pain-killers were effective. *I* didn't, but people weren't prepared to believe it or accept that.
Interviewer	Is there anything else you would like to tell me?
Respondent	It's hard to think at the moment. I'm sure there are lots of things I would love to say, but memory is beginning to fade now and all the things I thought of immediately I came out are beginning to die down. One thing I could perhaps mention is the complete feeling of helplessness a patient has when in hospital. The layman simply doesn't realize what's going on. Doctors and nurses are so all-powerful and you are totally at their mercy while you are in. I remember lying there feeling that I had absolutely no power to do anything on my own. I was so totally dependent on doctors and nurses that I don't think perhaps they realize just how the patient sees them and how much in awe patients are likely to be of them. It's hard to explain. I think it may be fear, the fact that you are lying there and you cannot do anything for yourself. You know at any given time a doctor can order this or a nurse can say that and it will be done *without* you having any notion of *why* it's being done and *what* good it's going to do or how *painful* it's going to be. I think that's the main thing really, the fact that you are *totally* dependent on the

nursing and medical staff or surgery staff whichever it may be.

Interviewer Were you happy to be dependent on them?

Respondent Oh no, no, no. I would have been initially, I assume but, as I say, having gone through these various days of pain, it suddenly came home to me that I really couldn't do anything but accept what was being done or not being done because I had no way of forcing my wishes on anyone or of explaining. I had to accept what was prescribed and what was said and all the rest of it.

Interviewer Did you feel that you were treated as a person, as an individual, or are you saying that you didn't?

Respondent Eventually. But while I was feeling very ill, no, not really. A body in a bed that had to be given this and that. You were treated very much like a child in lots of ways. Sisters tend to talk down to a patient, definitely. Doctors are a bit better but the sisters talk down to you. Maybe it's the way I speak to my children sometimes when they ask for something which I feel is quite impossible, but I usually give them an explanation as to why it is quite impossible whereas in hospital you are simply told, 'No, that can't be done'. That's it, without any reasonable explanation of why it can't be done.

Interviewer Anything else you would like to add?

Respondent Oh, one thing I found, yes, I must admit I remember this. After the operation you are expected to cough and bring up sputum. I have never been able to bring up sputum, I don't know why, even when I have a terrible cold I can't. But instead of being helped, I was told by sister that I would end up with pneumonia and a chest infection and, when I was lying there just longing for it all to be over, the thought of adding a chest infection and being in for so much longer was so depressing I could have burst into tears. It was left to the physiotherapist to reassure me that when my tubes had been taken out I would find it so much easier to cough and that there was no problem. I did not have to bring up sputum, I simply had to cough enough to move it around. According to the sister, I was heading for bronchopneumonia if I couldn't bring up sputum and I was very upset at that point because I felt I had another thing on top of the one I already had. Oh, it was horrifying. I could see days stretching ahead with me adding one illness on top of another without ever any way of improving the situation. So that was one point I remember, feeling very depressed one afternoon having been told this by sister, just two or three days after the operation and before I asked the physiotherapist. When the physiotherapist came she explained things so clearly that I realized it was nothing to get panicky about. But I had been told, 'You either bring up sputum or you end up with a chest infection, one or the other'. There was no choice and I was going mad trying to bring up sputum and just not succeeding. I actually got screens put round my bed one visiting hour so that I could continue trying without being in full view of visitors and patients. Terrible, it was really frightening that. As it is you are feeling very low and very much in pain and the thought of getting some other kind of illness on top of it – oh. So that was a particularly low day I remember during the time I was in.

Interviewer And you didn't really feel that the sister was particularly helpful?

Respondent Wasn't helpful at all. You shouldn't menace someone who is already feeling down, it's no help at all. I'd say *gentle encouragement*, which is what physiotherapists tend to provide. They got an awful lot more results, definitely. You always feel weepy anyway when you can't eat and you can't do this and you can't do that, but to be threatened with another illness is certainly not the way to improve the matter. I remember feeling particularly resentful towards that particular sister ever after.

Interviewer Anything else you would like to add?

Respondent No, I think that's about it.

Interviewer Thanks very much indeed. Thank you for letting me come and for telling me your experiences.

It is always a sobering experience to hear a patient's views. Several points brought out in the interview highlight the many myths about pain and lack of knowledge among nursing staff, in particular the individual nature of pain and the importance of believing a patient who says he is in pain, together with the issues of accountability and communication in relation to nursing practice. The above account is one of tragic mismanagement of one individual's pain. Of course, this does not happen to every patient but, when it does, it can result in serious emotional difficulties, particularly if subsequent hospitalization is required. After the interview, the patient said, 'I'm glad I've got it off my chest. I can concentrate on getting well again now'.

Research findings support some of the issues raised by the above experiences. Dodson (1985) suggested that attitudes of nursing and medical staff, the expression of pain by other patients, and the ward environment influence a person's response to pain. Sofaer (1984) found that in a sample of 64 nurses interviewed, 75% admired patients with will power, and 80% held the view that patients sometimes exaggerate pain. Seers (1989) more recently found that 43% of patients who had undergone elective abdominal surgery reported 'quite a lot of pain' or more on the first day after surgery. Twenty-two percent of patients rated their pain as 'very bad'. With regard to the fear of addiction, Cartwright (1985) found that 26% of nurses interviewed (n = 302) had reservations regarding opioid addiction, and only 7% said they would give injections for as long as a patient required them.

References

Cartwright, P. D. (1985) Pain control after surgery: a survey of current practice. *Annals of the Royal College of Surgeons of England*, 67:13–16.

Dodson, M. E. (1985) *The Management of Postoperative Pain*, Edward Arnold: London, pp. 21–50.

Seers, K. (1989) Patients' perception of acute pain. In *Directions in Nursing Research* (eds J. Wilson-Barnett and S. Robinson), pp. 107–16. Scutari Press: London.

Sofaer, B. (1984) *The Effect of Focused Education for Nursing Teams on Post-operative Pain of Patients*. Unpublished PhD thesis, University of Edinburgh.

2

Towards an understanding of pain

Pain is what the patient says it is and exists when he says it does.

(After McCaffery, 1983)

Meeting the challenge of pain control

Several disciplines in the fields of science, medicine, and the behavioural sciences have made valuable contributions towards the study of pain in recent years. These contributions have improved understanding of the nature of pain and of the various treatments available for pain relief. For example, neurophysiologists have studied how the nervous system reacts to painful stimuli, pharmacologists have been interested in developing more effective analgesic drugs, and psychologists have worked towards clarifying man's behaviour in relation to pain. Despite these and other efforts to meet the challenge of pain control, countless people still suffer unrelieved pain. Pain is the source of much misery in people's lives and the cause of much time spent off work.

Defining pain

The perception of, and response to, pain are the results of complex interactions of many factors. For this reason there are difficulties in trying to define pain. People who care for patients in pain must appreciate that they are dealing with a wide range of biological and behavioural differences which it may not be possible to explain in any one way, and that pain and injury are not necessarily related.

The following two definitions of pain allow for its subjective nature:

Pain is a complex phenomenon, a signal of tissue damage threat, an integrated defence reaction and a private experience of hurt

(Sternbach 1968)

and

> Pain is an unpleasant sensory and emotional experience associated with actual or potential tissue damage or described in terms of such damage. (The International Association for the Study of Pain Subcommittee on Taxonomy, 1979)

However, as far as nurses are concerned, because we have the most frequent contact with patients, an operational definition may be helpful and appropriate. The following definition is adapted from McCaffery (1983):

> Pain is what the patient says it is and exists when he says it does.

We cannot feel what the patient feels, yet it is not uncommon to overhear staff making comments that indicate that they disbelieve a patient. It is important to recognize that every patient is different. An additional problem for patients suffering pain (particularly chronic pain) is that the different specialists who may see and treat them have different perspectives of the same condition. The neurologist may talk of nerve pathways, and the psychologist of the emotional aspects of the pain experience; each specialist perhaps not fully appreciating aspects of a patient's condition that do not fall within his own area of specialization.

It is most important that those who care for patients in pain have a multidisciplinary outlook (Finer, 1980). This does not mean that nurses must be expert medical and behavioural scientists, only that they should be aware of the complex nature of each patient's pain and of the fact that relief can only be effective if the treatment (or combination of treatments) is aimed at controlling all the factors involved.

Placebo response

The placebo effect is thought to be due to suggestion, the wish to please the medical or nursing staff, or the patients belief that something is being done. Melzack and Wall (1982) revealed that the greater the suggestion that pain will be relieved, the greater the relief obtained by the patient. In addition, they revealed that in certain circumstances placebos are more effective for severe pain than for mild pain.

McCaffery (1983) defined placebo as 'any medical treatment that produces an effect in a patient because of its implicit or explicit therapeutic intent, and not because of its specific nature'. It is important to understand that because people are helped by placebos one should not imply that they do not suffer real acute or chronic pain, for no one can deny the reality of that pain.

Types of pain

Superficial, deep, and referred pain

Superficial pain involves the skin or mucous membranes. Superficial pain, which is thought to be transmitted by rapidly conducting A fibres, is perceived as distinct, sharp, well-defined pain, and can be described as bright, pricking, or burning. The nerve receptors of superficial (or cutaneous) pain are many, and can be activated by various stimuli. These may be mechanical, electrical, chemical, or thermal in nature.

Deep pain originating within the body is thought to be transmitted by thin, slow conducting C fibres. This type of pain may not be well localized, and usually has aching and diffuse qualities. Nerve receptors in the various organs are more widely spread than those of the skin. Stretching or tension may produce severe deep pain. In both superficial and deep pain, impulses are transmitted by pain fibres running in the sensory nerves to the posterior root ganglia of the spinal cord, and from there to the cortex, where they are interpreted as painful.

The impulses of referred pain also travel to the cortex, where they are interpreted as painful, but pain is felt at a site other than that which has been stimulated. However, the stimulated site and that at which pain is felt are invariably supplied by the same or an adjacent nerve. For example, the fallopian tubes have referred pain in the shoulders, and the appendix has referred pain in the region of the umbilicus.

The gate-control theory of pain

The gate-control theory of pain, developed by Melzack and Wall (1965), attempts to explain the variation in perception of identical stimulation. The theory relies upon complex neurophysiological processes. Put simply, the idea is that there is a 'gate' in the spinal cord, which under certain circumstances allows nerve impulses resulting from pain stimulation to pass through it and to be felt (interpreted by the brain). When the gate is 'open' pain impulses can flow through easily; when the gate is 'closed' none can pass through. It is thought that the degree of opening of the gate may in part be influenced via connections with the central nervous system, thus explaining the effect of psychological factors, such as anxiety, on pain perception.

Although the theory has evoked controversy among both scientists and clinicians, it has done away with the idea that pain is simply a sensation transmitted by nerves to a pain centre in the brain, and it provides a conceptual framework for the integration of the sensory, emotional, and behavioural dimensions of pain. This has implications for the treatment of pain using combinations of physical and psychological therapies.

The reader may wish to acquire useful background knowledge of the functional anatomy and physiology of pain, the development of pain theories, and the gate control theory in particular. Two recommended sources for such information are Francis (1987) and Latham (1990).

Acute and chronic pain

There are several areas where nurses have to face different problems in relation to pain management. Acute pain and chronic pain are different entities and must be treated differently. Management also varies according to patients' individual requirements.

Acute pain

Acute pain is pain that has a sudden onset and a foreseeable end. It is accompanied by fight-or-flight features such as dilation of pupils of the eyes, increased sweating, and increased pulse and respiration rate. Nurses encounter patients in acute pain in casualty departments, surgical wards and intensive care units. There are many techniques and drugs available for the relief of acute pain, but, nevertheless, there is much room for improvement in their application. For example, postoperative pain is often suffered unnecessarily. This may be due to shortage of trained nursing staff (Campbell, 1977). Allied to this is the fact that the protocol for drawing up and administering intramuscular opioids is complicated and time-consuming. Delays may result in patients experiencing unrelieved pain (Nayman, 1980). As well, prescribing habits of doctors could be improved (Cartwright, 1985). The personality factors discussed in Chapter 3 may add to the difficulties encountered. Furthermore, even if analgesics are prescribed to be given whenever necessary, patients may not be aware that pain relief is accessible (Campbell, 1977).

Acute trauma

The need for pain relief varies with the site of injury. Abdominal injuries and long bone fractures cause the most pain, whereas head and chest injuries give the least (Clarke, 1977).

It is of interest to consider two categories of patient who have suffered acute trauma, wounded soldiers and civilian casualties. There are important differences in the way these groups react to injury (Beecher,

1956). Soldiers may not report pain because they are relieved to be away from the battle area and pleased to find themselves alive. The civilian casualty, on the other hand, may feel very resentful, particularly if his injury occurred because of someone else's carelessness. Such a patient may need sedation as well as analgesia.

Chronic pain

Chronic pain is more of a 'situation', whereas acute pain can be regarded as an 'event' (Twycross and Lack, 1983). Nurses encounter chronic pain particularly in medical wards and during home care. Its management presents many problems, particularly because of the effect it has on the lifestyle of people who suffer it. It is important to distinguish between chronic pain of non-malignant origin and cancer pain.

Chronic pain of non-malignant origin may be accompanied by sleep disturbances, loss of appetite and libido, constipation, preoccupation with the illness, changes in personality, and inability to work. The approach to managing this pain has to be flexible and may possibly involve combinations of several treatments such as transcutaneous electric nerve stimulation, acupuncture and/or relaxation therapy (Chapter 7). It is important to realize that chronic pain such as sciatica, low-back pain and postherpetic neuralgia are not life threatening, although the quality of a person's life is altered by having pain (Lipton, 1979).

Care must be taken in the prescribing of opioid analgesic drugs as some patients may be likely to develop dependence. Some non-opioid medications may be useful in reducing the level of pain. An important aspect to consider when dealing with patients suffering chronic pain of non-malignant origin is the process of adaptation. Somehow, some individuals may manage to endure pain and carry on despite it. They may appear untroubled and may get through their work by means of sheer willpower, although there may be accompanying signs of depression. Staff may then, erroneously, be more concerned with the apparent depression than with the underlying unexpressed pain which is its cause. Walker *et al.* (1989) suggested that when pain cannot be cured or eliminated, as is often the case with sufferers of chronic pain, the patient must learn to cope with, or gain control over, the pain, and in so doing may need help.

Cancer pain is managed differently from chronic pain of non-malignant origin. There is a need for carers to be aware that open communication between nurses, patients and doctors will be of help to patients in living their last days free from fear and anxiety. With cancer, one is dealing with a process of progressive change. It is important to review pain relief regularly because the pattern of pain may change. All aspects of body and mind comfort should be attended to. With cancer pain, patients may have both the fight-or-flight reactions normally associated with acute pain as well as insomnia, lack of appetite and loss of libido, constipation, personality changes, preoccupation with symptoms and lack of interest in work. If cancer pain is not controlled, patients become very demoralized and wearied by suffering. Good management of cancer pain seeks to support the cancer patient by provision of adequate medication, rest and attention (Twycross and Lack, 1983).

Wherever the nurse finds herself caring for patients in pain, be it in areas of acute care or in the management of chronic or terminal pain, it is important that she is constantly aware that pain is what the patient says it is, and exists when he says it does. Judgemental attitudes, disbelief, and withholding pain relief are not helpful when 'it hurts'.

Some problems faced by nurses in managing pain

When asked about problems they faced in trying to help patients in pain, groups of nurses identified the following difficulties.

For patients with acute pain:

- Lack of awareness among nursing staff of severity of patients' pain.
- Fear among nurses of masking symptoms by analgesia.
- Acceptance of analgesia regime without seeking alternatives.
- Lack of recording of patients' pain.
- Ignorance of drug efficacies.
- Problems of communication between nurses, patients and doctors.

For patients with chronic pain:

- Referrals to several different specialists or doctors resulting in patients being given different and sometimes conflicting explanations and/or information.
- Coping with patients' depression, anxiety, and hostility in general wards.
- Helping patients to cope with life.
- Physical manifestations of pain may not be present.
- Frustration among staff.
- Problems of communication between patients and staff.

For patients terminally ill at home:

- Helping the patient to cope.
- Educating relatives and helping them to cope.
- Communication between nursing staff and the general practitioner.
- Difficulties of liaison with hospital.

For patients terminally ill in hospital:

- Lack of privacy for the patient.
- Ignorance among staff regarding pain control.
- Problems of communication between patients, relatives, nurses and doctors.

It is not within the scope of this book to cover all the points mentioned above. However, an awareness by nurses that these problems exist will go some way towards facing the challenge of pain control.

Summary

- Several disciplines have contributed to the study of pain, yet many people suffer unrelieved pain.
- Pain is a complex subjective phenomenon. It is important to realize that everyone is different.
- A definition of pain appropriate for nursing is 'pain is what the patient says it is and exists when he says it does'.
- There are three types of pain: superficial, deep, and referred.
- The gate-control theory of pain attempts to explain the variation in perception of identical stimulation.
- Acute pain and chronic pain are different entities, and their management is therefore different.
- Judgemental attitudes by nurses are not helpful to patients when 'it hurts'.
- Nurses themselves are able to identify several problems when caring for patients in pain.

References

Beecher, H. K. (1956) Relationship of significance of wound to pain experienced, *Journal of the American Medical Association*, 161:1609–13.
Campbell, D. (1977) The management of post-operative pain, Chapter 13, in *Pain: New Perspectives in Measurement and Management* (eds A. W. Harcus, R. Smith and B. Whittle), Churchill Livingstone, London and Edinburgh.

Cartwright, P. D. (1985) Pain control after surgery: a survey of current practice. *Annals of the Royal College of Surgeons of England*, 67:13–16.

Clarke, R. S. (1977) The analgesic management of acute trauma, Chapter 14, in *Pain: New Perspectives in Measurement and Management* (eds A. W. Harcus, R. Smith and B. Whittle), Churchill Livingstone, London and Edinburgh.

Finer, B. (1980) Hypnotherapy, Chapter 2, in *Persistent Pain* (ed. S. Lipton), Vol. 2, Academic Press, London.

Francis, I. W. (1987) The Physiology of Pain in *Nursing the Physically Ill Adult* (eds J. R. P. Boore, R. Champion and M. C. Ferguson), Churchill Livingstone, Edinburgh.

International Association for the Study of Pain Subcommittee on Taxonomy (1979) Pain terms: A list with definitions and notes on usage, *Pain*, 6:249–52.

Latham, J. (1990) *Pain Control*. Austen Cornish Ltd with The Lisa Sainsbury Foundation.

Lipton, S. (1979) The treatment of chronic pain, Chapter 10, in *The Control of Chronic Pain* (ed. S. Lipton), Edward Arnold.

McCaffery, M. (1983) *Nursing the Patient in Pain*, Harper & Row.

Melzack, R. and Wall, P. D. (1965) Pain mechanisms: A new theory, *Science*, 150:971–9.

Melzack, R. and Wall, P. D. (1982) *The Challenge of Pain*, Penguin Books.

Nayman, J. (1980) Control of postoperative pain: A multidisciplinary approach, in *Problems in Pain: Proceedings of the First Australia–New Zealand Conference on Pain* (eds C. Peck and M. Wallace), Pergamon Press.

Sternbach, R. A. (1968) *Pain: A Psychophysiological Analysis*, Academic Press.

Twycross, R. G. and Lack, S. A. (1983) *Symptom Control in Far Advanced Cancer Pain Relief*, Pitman.

Walker, J. M., Akinsanya, J. A., Davis, B. D. and Marcer, D. (1989) The nursing management of pain in the community: a theoretical framework. *Journal of Advanced Nursing*, 14:240–7.

3

The uniqueness of the individual

The evidence shows that pain is much more variable and modifiable than many people have believed in the past. Pain differs from person to person, culture to culture.

(After Melzack and Wall, 1982)

Psychological factors

There is no predictable relationship between pain and injury. Each individual's pain experience is influenced by his unique personal history, by the meaning he attaches to his pain, and by his state of mind. People with the same or similar conditions will behave differently because of variation in background and personality. It is important for nurses to recognize this and to realize the crucial part that psychology plays in behaviour during illness.

Many nurses and health carers think that they, not the patient, can decide whether or not pain exists, and if it does, how intense it is. Taylor et al. (1983), in a study on hypothetical patients, found that nurses attributed less pain to patients who had no obvious signs of pathology, or who were suffering from long-term pain. Some nurses may feel uneasy about believing a patient's statements about pain, but since we have no objective evidence for the diagnosis and treatment of pain, we must rely solely on the patient to tell us what he feels and whether the treatment is effective.

Sometimes patients adapt to pain both physiologically and behaviourally so that it is not easy for carers to see if a patient is suffering. Minimal expressions of pain may therefore be misunderstood. Sometimes the cause of pain may not be easy to identify and a patient's pain may be erroneously dismissed by staff. But we must accept that all pain is real, regardless of its cause, and that most bodily pain probably results from a combination of physical and psychological factors.

A knowledge of psychological factors associated with pain will be helpful to the nurse in understanding patients' reactions. Areas of psychology that are particularly relevant are personality characteristics and the relationship of anxiety and depression to pain. Anxiety is particularly associated with acute pain, and depression with chronic pain.

Personality characteristics

Personality is the unique mix of intellectual and emotional qualities that each person reflects in his behaviour. It is helpful to know what a patient's personality was like prior to the onset of a painful illness or injury so that his behaviour or changes in behaviour can be understood. Pain is often regarded merely as a symptom of physical or mental illness. It is important that nurses deal with pain from both the physical and the psychological standpoints.

The influence of personality on people's pain tolerance and pain thresholds has been studied by many researchers. In general, pain thresholds have been found to be lower for introverted people than for extroverts, but extroverts have tended to report pain more freely. In one study, it was found that extrovert subjects received more analgesia than introvert subjects (Bond and Pearson, 1969). In terms of emotionality, those who are most emotional have the most pain (Bond, 1979).

Extroversion and emotionality can be assessed using formal psychological testing, although it is not usual practice to do this for patients on routine admission to general hospitals. Even when using such testing, it may not be possible to identify with certainty those who will have the most pain (Parbrook et al., 1973).

It may be helpful though, to both staff and patients, for a nurse to ask each patient on admission how he sees himself in terms of personality. It can be useful for staff to have a record on the care plan of how each patient usually reacts to illness and stress, and his attitude to this particular admission. It is helpful for the patient to know that staff are aware of how he normally copes with pain. It should also be made clear to patients at this time what provisions will be made for pain relief. Staff take it for granted that they will provide some sort of analgesia, but patients like to know. If nothing else, it lets the patient know that staff are interested in him as a person and in his well-being, before, during, and after a potentially painful event. This knowledge alone can have a pronounced effect in reducing anxiety, particularly in overanxious people whose fear may be based, among other things, on the fear of pain itself.

Anxiety

Most people become apprehensive when faced with a painful illness. Those who tend to be worriers by nature, when confronted by such an event may become so anxious that they are overwhelmed. For these patients, pain may be greater because pain causes anxiety (particularly acute pain) and anxiety, in turn, may heighten pain perception.

It has been reported that preparing a patient in advance for surgery by giving information and by teaching coping techniques may help (Johnson et al., 1970). In addition, research by Hayward (1975), Boore (1977), and Davis (1988) have shown that in terms of anxiety reduction and consequent decreased postoperative pain, it may benefit patients to have preoperative information. Fear of the unknown may compound the pain experience. The patient in pain may have lost self-esteem; information may give them insight. The underlying idea is that, if a person can understand better what to expect, this understanding will reduce his anxiety and, in turn, his pain. However, it is important to know something about the patient's feelings in relation to his normal anxiety level. A moderately anxious person may do a little 'worry work' which can be helpful in building up psychological defences to deal with the stress, but those whose normal anxiety level is either very high or very low may be at a disadvantage (Janis, 1958). An overanxious individual may find difficulty in developing the inner strength to cope, whereas a very calm person may be quite disagreebly surprised by the inescapable stress and pain. Self-medication often helps patients to feel in control of the situation.

As far as nursing implications are concerned, it is important to try to identify what information would be helpful to individual patients as part of preparation for surgery or other potentially painful events. It should be noted, however, that the mental and emotional state of a patient can vary with time, and that this may have an effect on severity, tolerance and expression of pain.

Pain may be seen unconsciously by patients as punishment, as a symbol of rejection or as a way of asking for help. Just as it may be a warning to the body, so it may be interpreted as a warning to the personality. Most often, pain is perceived as a threat to body image, producing anxiety. The nurse must be aware of signs of anxiety which may manifest as restlessness, avoidance of discussion or hostility (sometimes labelled as uncooperativeness). The nurse should respond with kindness and understanding to such situations, as defensiveness may increase a patient's stress.

Depression

Some people respond to stress by feeling a little low, while others feel a sense of despair. Patients in pain, particularly those who experience chronic pain and have had their lives altered by their inability to function socially, and by difficulties with the activities of daily living, may experience considerable depression. Obviously, if a person normally has a tendency to feel low he will be more likely to suffer despair as a result of chronic pain. Coping with pain becomes even more difficult in these circumstances. Wade *et al.* (1990) suggested that anger and frustration are also important components of the emotional unpleasantness suffered by people with chronic pain. It is important for nurses to be aware of these factors when supporting patients.

Other psychological factors

People who have a tendency towards hysterical, hypochondriac, or obsessional behaviour may respond to pain in a variety of ways which can bring them into conflict with medical or nursing staff. This may present problems, especially when staff expect patients to conform to an expected pattern of behaviour. Sometimes colleagues use the term 'supratentorial' when referring to patients whose pain they may not believe has a physical basis. The use of this term may be a way of avoiding clear thinking, and is used for any pain the speaker does not feel is 'justified' – anything from conversion hysteria to an extreme reaction to pain because of fear. Nurses should be aware of the use of this term, and guard against being taken in by it. The influence of personality on pain thresholds and tolerance has important implications for nursing care. Knowing that there is a relationship between personality and pain may help the nurse in her attempts to individualize care.

Another point of particular note when considering psychological factors is the influence of fatigue. With prolonged pain, the patient gets more tired and there is an accompanying lowering of pain threshold.

Psychogenic pain

Psychological factors play such an important part in pain perception and expression that sometimes a patient may be labelled as having pain which is 'psychogenic'. In such situations the patient is presumed to need or want pain. Such a patient may undergo several surgical operations and be seen by many different doctors but no organic basis may be found for recurrent pain. For the patient, however, the pain is real, and lack of relief, together with lack of understanding by carers, may lead to depression requiring psychotherapy. Sometimes family therapy may be helpful, especially if a patient 'uses' his pain to 'control' the family (Sternbach, 1970). Of course, in addition, during the process of undergoing unsuccessful treatments or operations, a person's body may incur scarring and/or adhesions which may add to his pain problem.

It is *most important* that the term 'psychogenic pain' is *reserved* for patients who have absolutely no physical finding and a definite psychological history that points in the direction of expressing emotional problems in terms of pain (Sternbach, 1982). It should be noted that for most patients experiencing chronic pain, the pain has an underlying physical basis, with emotional and behavioural factors contributing in varying degrees to the perception and expression of pain. It has been shown that it is more usual for a psychological disturbance to be the result of chronic pain rather than the cause of it, and that psychological manifestations may disappear after successful treatment of the pain (Sternbach and Timmermans, 1975).

Psychiatric illness

A number of psychiatric illnesses such as depression and schizophrenia have pain as a symptom. If the psychiatric illness is treated successfully, the pain will often disappear.

The effect of learning on pain

The role that psychology plays in the pain experience of an individual is a complex one, dependent on physical or psychiatric illness, early life experiences, present environment, the meaning he attaches to pain, and his cultural background. These factors add up to the learning experience which colours the patient's attitude towards his pain.

The reader might like to try the following exercise to illustrate the effect of learning on pain. Close your eyes for a few minutes and think back to your early childhood. Try to recall a situation where you experienced a painful event – perhaps you fell off your bike and hurt your knee, or you may have burnt your fingers in a pot of hot water. Recall if you can, the reaction of a person who was with you or near you at the time – was it panic, anger, love or ridicule? What action was taken? How did you feel afterwards? Try doing this recall with some of your nursing colleagues and compare experiences and reactions. Early experiences such as these, as well as parental behaviour, colour everybody's future attitude towards pain. Together, these experiences constitute a patient's 'pain autobiography'.

So it is with patients facing stressful events – each person has a different learning experience to bring to his own situation.

Modelling

One aspect of learning is known as modelling (Bandura, 1971). This refers to the idea that a person can anticipate the behavioural consequences of a situation through observing others, without having to experience it himself. Thus, he may subsequently base his reaction to his own experience on the behaviour of those he has observed. Patients may or may not express pain according to the social modelling that goes on in a ward. However, they do learn to lean on each other for support and for strategies of pain control. It is not uncommon for patients to say, 'Everybody is in the same boat'. Nevertheless, if a patient does not verbally express his pain and behaves as the 'social norms' of the ward dictate, it does not necessarily mean that his pain is being relieved.

Cultural factors

General observations of similarity in behaviour between members of the same ethnic group in relation to pain have led to the idea that cultural factors are an important consideration in the management of pain. In some cultures, rituals which we may associate with extreme discomfort seem to cause no trouble for the people involved, whereas in others, apparently trivial stimuli produce a marked response. Research has shown that pain tolerance levels do indeed vary from one cultural background to another (Sternbach and Tursky, 1965). For example, people of Anglo-Saxon origin tend to accept pain in a matter of fact way, whereas people with a Mediterranean background are more expressive of their pain (Zborowski, 1969). These reactions are closely related to early childhood experiences.

Our own culture tends to favour a high tolerance for pain, although, as in any cultural group, tolerance varies greatly from one patient to another and also in the same patient in different situations. For example, a patient may be willing to tolerate pain while his family is visiting so that he can communicate with them, but he is not willing to endure the same degree of pain at other times.

Some patients refuse pain relief because they have a high pain tolerance, whereas others are not willing to endure any pain for any period of time. Sometimes staff place a value judgement on a patient's tolerance without realizing that this is his own unique response to pain and that he is entitled to such a response. If a patient is a member of an ethnic minority, this could lead to unwarranted judgement of future patients from the same minority group. Such judgement would obstruct effective pain management.

The meaning of pain

There is also evidence to suggest that people attach meaning to their pain, which may influence the intensity and duration of the pain they feel and their readiness to accept or refuse medication. Some people may consider that the pain they are suffering is a form of punishment they must endure for past misdeeds, while others may say, 'What have I done to deserve this?' A patient may refuse drugs because he believes they are a crutch, thinking that succumbing to sickness is a sign of weakness, and that self-respect can be maintained by rejecting help (Amarasingham, 1980). Patients who believe in certain systems of values may be resistant to accepting advice. For example, Puerto Ricans in New York classified food, medicines, and bodily states according to whether they were hot or cold. Hot substances were used to treat cold conditions, and vice versa. Rashes and diarrhoea were considered hot and should therefore be treated with cool foods or medicines (Harwood, 1971).

Some suggestions for the psychological support of patients in pain

- Develop a relationship with a patient which gives the patient an opportunity to discuss his feelings.
- Try to find out from the patient how he sees himself in terms of personality. This will give you some clues as to how he may be helped to cope with stress and/or pain.
- Provide the patient with information about what he will experience in terms of hospital routines and procedures.
- Discuss with the patient how he feels about analgesia. For example, does he have any coping strategies of his own which he would like to try out? Emphasize the availability of pain relief as part of nursing care.
- Involve the patient as a *partner* in this effort and not as a *dependant*. In this way you will give him a sense of *control*. For the patient, this sense of control, both in aucte and chronic pain, will decrease pain intensity and improve the quality of the patient's life. Many psychological strategies taught to patients, such as relaxation, are aimed at giving the patient greater control over his pain. These are discussed in Chapter 7.

Allowing for individual variation

There is a great danger of stereotyping patients. Nurses *must* make allowances for individual variations in relation to pain expression and the response to various therapies. Above all, nurses must avoid labelling patients as 'good' or 'bad', 'co-operative' or 'unco-operative'. The world is made up of millions of unique individuals. We have to *accept* that there are innumerable combinations of personality, childhood experience and cultural background. Our response as nurses must be to individualize pain relief. This means accepting that the patient's pain is what he says it is (a unique perception of his unique physical and psychological self) and that it exists when he says it does. The individual nature of pain is described below in the exact words of a man who has had phantom-limb pain for 47 years:

> There is no method to accurately describe pain. Various words used such as, itch, tender, ache, discomfort, sore, agonizing, searing, burning, shooting, excruciating really convey little understanding to the listener. They may be understatements, exaggerations, or the wrong use of terms. Most phenomena have a common universal method of measurement, such as, sound, wind velocity, earthquake intensity, and so on. But no sufferer can tell a doctor how much pain he is suffering, nor can a doctor measure it. Assuming that a reliable method is made available, the next problem would be the effect of pain of the same intensity on different individuals. Some would be incapacitated with, say, a figure of four; others would be able to function.

Summary

- There is no predictable relationship between pain and injury.
- We must rely on the patient for reports of his pain and the effectiveness of treatment.
- Sometimes patients adapt to pain both physiologically and behaviourally.
- Personality characteristics influence pain tolerance and pain threshold.
- Anxiety is associated with acute pain and depression with chronic pain.
- Anxiety heightens pain perception.
- Preparing a patient in advance for surgery by giving him relevant information may reduce anxiety.
- Pain is fatiguing.
- The term 'psychogenic pain' must be reserved for patients with no physical findings and a history of psychological problems.
- Each person has a different learning experience to bring to his own painful situation.
- A patient's behaviour may be influenced by behaviour that he has observed in others.
- Cultural factors play an important part in pain expression.
- People attach different meanings to pain.

- Nurses should support patients psychologically by:
  - developing relationships;
  - finding out how the patients see themselves;
  - providing information;
  - discussing analgesia;
  - involving the patient in treatment.
- Nurses should allow for individual variation in response to pain and its treatment.

References

Amarasingham, L. R. (1980) Social and cultural perspectives on medication refusal, *American Journal of Psychiatry*, 137:353–8.

Bandura, A. (1971) Analysis of modeling processes, in *Psychological Modeling* (ed. A. Bandura), Aldine-Atherton.

Bond, M. R. (1979) *Pain: Its Nature Analysis and Treatment*, Churchill Livingstone.

Bond, M. R. and Pearson, I. B. (1969) Psychological aspects of pain in women with advanced cancer of the cervix, *Journal of Psychosomatic Research*, 13:13–19.

Boore, J. (1977) Preoperative care of patients. *Nursing Times* 73:12, 409–11.

Davis, P. S. (1988) Changing nursing practice for more effective control of post operative pain through a staff initiated educational programme. *Nurse Education Today* 8, 325–31.

Harwood, A. (1971) The hot-cold theory of disease: Implications for treatment of Puerto Rican patients, *Journal of the American Medical Association*, 216:1153–8.

Hayward, J. (1975) Information, a prescription against pain. *R.C.N. Research Series*.

Janis, I. L. (1958) *Psychological Stress*, Wiley.

Johnson, J. E., Dabbs, J. M. and Leventhall, H. (1970) Psychological factors in the welfare of surgical patients, *Nursing Research*, 19:18–29.

Melzack, R. and Wall, P. D. (1982) *The Challenge of Pain*, Penguin Books.

Parbrook, G. D., Dalrymple, D. G. and Steel, D. F. (1973) Personality assessment and postoperative pain and complications, *Journal of Psychosomatic Research*, 17:277–85.

Seers, K. (1989) Patients' perception of acute pain, in *Directions in Nursing Research* (eds J. Wilson-Barnett and S. Robinson), pp. 107–16, Scutari Press.

Sofaer, B. (1984) *The Effect of Focused Education for Nursing Teams on Post-operative Pain of Patients*. Unpublished PhD thesis, University of Edinburgh.

Sternbach, R. A. (1970) Strategies and tactics in the treatment of patients with pain, in *Pain and Suffering, Selected Aspects* (ed. B. L. Crue), Thomas Springfield.

Sternbach, R. A. (1982) The psychologists role in the diagnosis and treatment of pain patients, Chapter 1, in *Psychological Approaches to the Management of Pain* (eds J. Barber and C. Adrian), Brunner Mazal.

Sternbach, R. A. and Turskey, B. (1965) Ethnic differences in psychophysical and skin potential responses to electric shock. *Psychophysiology*, 1:241–6.

Sternbach, R. A. and Timmermans, G. (1975) Personality changes associated with reduction of pain, *Pain*, 1:177–81.

Taylor, A. G., Skelton, J. and Butcher, J. (1983) Duration of pain, condition and physical pathology: determinants of nurses' assessments of patients in pain. *Nursing Research*, 33, 4–8.

Wade, J., Price, D. D., Hamer, R. M., Schwartz, S. M. and Hart, R. P. (1990) An emotional component analysis of chronic pain. *Pain*, 40, 303–10.

Zborowski, M. (1969) *People in Pain*, Jossey-Bass Inc.

4

The unique position of the nurse

> I envy for our medical students the advantages enjoyed by the nurses who
> live in daily contact with the sick.
>
> (Osler, 1947)

Nurses, more than other health carers, have the opportunity to develop close and fulfilling relationships with patients. In this respect nurses are in a unique position to assess the physical and psychological well-being of patients, especially in response to treatment, and to communicate this information to each other, their medical colleagues, and other members of the caring team.

Nurses' own beliefs and values

As discussed in Chapter 3, a patient brings to each painful situation his past experiences of pain, experiences coloured not only by his own personality but by the behaviour of those around him at the time. However, the patient is not alone in bringing a pain autobiography to a current situation, since those who care for him also have pain autobiographies. In some situations this might be of help to a patient but in others it may not. For example, a nurse who has suffered pain herself is likely to have a greater understanding of a patient's pain than one who has not, while a nurse brought up to believe in a 'grin-and-bear-it' attitude towards pain might not find it easy to empathize with a patient.

A patient who comes into hospital is thus faced with a team of carers who may have different attitudes and values in relation to pain, its expression, and control. A key person in British hospital wards is the charge nurse, whose attitudes and beliefs influence whether or not a patient receives the best possible pain relief, firstly through her reports to the medical staff about the patient and, secondly, because of her responsibility and power in relation to interpreting administration times for drugs or other therapies. Again the danger is one of interpreting a patient's needs in accordance with set routines or inbuilt personal values about pain, whereas, of course, patients' needs are as individual as they themselves are, and pain relief should be administered accordingly. Unfortunately, however, research findings have shown that nurses and patients may lack agreement about the severity of patient's pain (Seers, 1989). Sofaer (1984) found that only 9% of nurses (n = 64) felt that the aim of administering analgesics during the first two postoperative days was to relieve pain completely, compared with 28% of patients (n = 87).

Personal judgements

Nurses may make personal judgements of patients' suffering based on their own beliefs. The following extract is quoted from Davitz and Davitz★ and illustrates how feelings and behaviour were affected as a result of personal judgements:

> On the unit, she [the nurse] attended two mothers. One had a normal healthy baby girl and the other gave birth to a boy with a cleft palate. Both mothers reacted negatively to the births. The mother of the baby girl had wanted a boy. She was hysterical, refused to see the infant, and became withdrawn and hostile. The mother of the baby with a cleft palate displayed equally violent reactions. She, too, rejected all contact with the infant and staff. The nurse reacted to the mother of the baby who had a cleft palate with great sympathy and understanding. 'I went in to see her and no matter what she said or did, I knew I had to stay and help. She needed us, though she fought against all the help we tried to give'. The mother of the girl received routine care. 'It drove us up a wall to hear this woman carrying on the way she did. She was lucky she had a healthy baby. For her to complain didn't make sense. All of us could understand the feelings of the woman who had a baby with a cleft palate – but this woman kind of made us angry. None of us felt like rushing in to see her when she called.'
>
> Each of the patients felt distressed. From the mothers' points of view, the psychological strain of the disappointing births might have been comparable. However, from the nurse's point of view the situations differed. The two women simply weren't seen as suffering the same degree of psychological distress. The nurse's reactions were not determined by differences in the behaviour of the two women. As a matter of fact, the two mothers apparently behaved in very much the same way. Thus, it was not the patients' behaviour that made the difference, but the nurse's beliefs about suffering. She didn't believe that the mother who was disappointed with the sex of her baby could suffer as much as the mother of a baby born with a cleft palate. The crucial difference in the matter, therefore, was the nurse's system of beliefs about suffering.

★ In *RN, The Full-Service Nursing Journal.* 1975 © Medical Economics Company Inc., Oradell, NJ. Reprinted with permission.

The same authors studied nurses' inferences of suffering by asking nurses to rate the degree of physical pain and degree of psychological distress of patients suffering from 15 different illnesses and injuries. They found that nurses have some common beliefs about suffering:

Results show that a patient's socio-economic status, age, and ethnic background are important determinants of the amount of suffering likely to be inferred by a nurse. For example, lower-class patients were generally seen as suffering greater physical pain than middle or upper-class patients. For instance, an unskilled labourer with thrombophlebitis was seen as experiencing greater pain than either a teacher or bank president of the same age and sex. Nurses saw male and female patients suffering equivalent degrees of physical pain and psychological distress. However, when sex was considered in relationship to social class, the fact that a patient was male or female did make a difference. For example, lower-class women were seen as suffering more physical pain than lower-class men who had the same illnesses or injuries and were the same age. However, the reverse was true for upper-class women and men. Upper-class women were seen as suffering *less* physical pain than upper-class men. . . . Ethnic background of the patient also influences the degree of inferred suffering. Among six ethnic groups considered (Jewish, Black, Oriental, Mediterranean, Anglo-Saxon/Teutonic and Spanish), Jewish patients were consistently rated as having the greatest physical pain and the greatest psychological distress. Spanish patients were second; Anglo-Saxon/Teutonic and Oriental the lowest. Thus, regardless of age, diagnosis, or social class background, Jewish patients were seen as suffering significantly more pain and psychological distress than other patients.

The researchers concluded that it is important to recognize that belief systems about suffering exist because these systems have a potential influence on interactions between patients and nurses insofar as nurses may have preconceived notions or expectations regarding the pain and psychological distress of patients. Davitz and Davitz also reported an instance where one nurse mentioned her reaction to an Oriental patient who was crying in a casualty department. The nurse had observed stoicism in Oriental patients previously, and felt taken aback when she was confronted with someone who did not fulfil her expectations.

Another study has shown that nurses were less responsive to men than to women patients in terms of reports about their pain (Pilowsky and Bond, 1969). Men rated their pain as more severe and asked for pain relief more often, but nurses actually gave them less medication than the women. There was an expectation by the nurses that pain should be tolerated more by men than by women. One explanation is that since most nurses are women, they are more able to identify with other women. However, some nurses may feel the opposite – that women exaggerate pain, therefore it may be easier to believe men. We all have our own beliefs, but we must be *aware* that we may be wrong and so avoid imposing our values on patients.

On the other hand, bringing prior knowledge (rather than prejudice) to a situation may be helpful. For example, if a certain illness is usually very painful, then the nurse can be on the look-out for signs of distress. Nevertheless, as already pointed out, we should be aware of the dangers of stereotyping because it can lead to misunderstandings. It is important that nurses examine their own beliefs and values about suffering and learn to be on their guard for misperceptions and misunderstandings.

Incongruence of beliefs and values within the caring team

It is not uncommon for members of the caring team to disagree on how best to provide pain relief for a particular patient. It is sometimes found that the more junior staff are more compassionate towards patients, but unfortunately also the most powerless. The following anecdote, from the interview reported in Chapter 1, illustrates this point. The student nurses knew the patient was in pain and were sympathetic. They reported the patient's pain to the charge nurse, who came and said, 'This is *not* the time to take pain-killers. Pain-killers are given out at certain times and you certainly shouldn't have any need of them at this point in the day.' The patient felt that pain did not come very high on the list of priorities. Washing people, changing beds and keeping things clean seemed to be regarded as more important, at least to those with authority.

The patient who is in pain just wants relief. Nurses who are not in a position to sanction relief, or request review of analgesic requirements by the doctor because of their lack of seniority, can be made to feel helpless and stressed. It is not uncommon for junior nurses to apologize to patients by saying something like, 'I'm afraid you're not due your pain killers yet', or 'The drug trolley will be around in half an hour'. If a patient reports pain to a nurse before the time when medication is due according to the prescription, then the nurse in charge *must* consider it her responsibility to inform the doctor with a view to increasing the efficacy of the medication. Doctors rely on nursing colleagues to report patients' pain because they themselves cannot be on hand 24 hours a day to assess with the patient his individual requirements (Chapter 6).

Responses to and expectations of patients' behaviour

Sometimes nurses' concern about a patient's distress is related to the medical diagnosis or to the type of operation the patient has had. For example, pain following minor surgery may be dismissed because of the simplicity of the surgical technique involved, whereas someone who has undergone a more complicated surgical procedure may evoke more attention. The nurse, without paying attention to what the patient himself is experiencing, may feel that the latter type of operation should result in more pain. One ex-patient, herself a nurse, reported pain in her chest to the nursing staff on her admission to hospital. No pain relief or sympathy was forthcoming until a diagnosis had been made.

Illnesses or procedures have different meanings for different people, and these may affect their pain behaviour. Someone, for example, may be so relieved at undergoing a hysterectomy following years of unpleasant symptoms that the postoperative pain may be much better tolerated than that experienced by a patient who has undergone another form of surgery but who has had no previous symptoms. Nurses should therefore not have rigid expectations of the way a patient with a given condition should feel. For example, it is not helpful to make remarks such as, 'Mrs Jones had the same operation two days ago and she is up and about', or, prior to a procedure, 'You should be up and about in 24 hours'. If patients have difficulty in meeting these expectations they may feel a sense of failure.

Prejudice on the part of the nurse may be related to patient adaptation. In this situation a patient's pain may be less socially visible and the patient is consequently regarded with suspicion. Hackett (1971), a psychiatrist interested in treating patients in pain, has written:

> The individual stands before you in the examining room calmly and coolly describing the agony he is in and your first response is to doubt that he suffers as much as he claims.

It is important to remember that whereas the patient may have adapted his behaviour, the pain may remain at the same intensity.

In relation to painful procedures, sometimes nurses say, 'You won't feel anything', or 'This will hurt a little', or 'It shouldn't be *that* sore'. It would be more helpful to patients if the nurse said something along the following lines: 'This may be painful for some people – let me know how it is for you'. In this way, the patient is not embarrassed into conforming with the nurse's expectations of him and is allowed to express *his* own experience.

One difficulty often voiced by nurses is in assessing the efficacy of analgesic drugs. If a patient reports pain prior to the time when the next dose of medication is due, he should not be made to feel that he is reacting in an inappropriate way. There is much evidence, particularly in relation to relief of postoperative pain, to suggest that undertreatment of patients is alarmingly common (Marks and Sachar, 1973; Cohen, 1980; Weis *et al.*, 1983). A patient's behaviour should *not* be thoughtlessly compared to that of other patients who have undergone the same or similar operations.

Both the efficacy and duration of action of a drug can vary from one patient to another. This problem is often compounded by standard prescriptional frameworks such as the 'magic' four-hourly regime. Nurses often expect patients' behaviour to conform to this regime. Sometimes, if patients manage to conform, they are labelled 'awfully good' as if they do not, they are labelled as 'unco-operative' or 'complaining'. One staff nurse said, 'Before I learnt about the individual nature of pain, I classified patients according to their operations and expected them to behave alike in relation to their pain relief requirements.'

Learning about pain relief

It may be worth digressing here to comment on this staff nurse's remarks. Perhaps the most significant factor contributing to lack of awareness of the importance of pain relief among health carers is the lack of education on the subject of pain and its relief in student curricula. Since man's fear of pain is associated with his fear of death (Sternbach, 1968), this lamentable situation must be remedied both during basic training and by postbasic continuing education programmes. Lack of education could be a primary problem faced by nursing staff when trying to help patients in pain. Sofaer (1984) found that 14% of nurses felt themselves to be well prepared, 75% would have liked more education, and 11% felt themselves to be badly prepared. Trained nurses act as models for less experienced nurses. If trained staff are poorly informed on current research and theory in relation to pain and its relief, then the *status quo* of lack of knowledge and ill-founded myths will continue. One staff nurse commented, 'For years I've been handing out analgesics, never thinking about whether they were effective or not or how long they lasted.'

If a nurse *is* well informed on aspects of pain management, however, she could use the combination of her unique position as a carer, together with her knowledge, to increase her own confidence. She would be placed in a better position then to exercise professional accountability and responsibility, themes that are becoming generally accepted principles in nursing. These themes are discussed in the next chapter.

Summary

- Nurses are in a unique position to communicate with patients, each other and medical staff.
- There is a danger of nurses interpreting a patient's needs in accordance with their own inbuilt personal values about pain.

- Incongruence of beliefs and values within a caring team may not be helpful to the patient in pain.
- Routine drug round administrations may not meet the needs of patients who suffer pain.
- Staff may have expectations of a patient's pain response to a particular disease or procedure.
- Even if a patient adapts to pain it may remain at the same intensity.
- The efficacy and duration of action of a drug can vary from one patient to another.
- Being well-informed about pain management will increase a nurse's confidence.

References

Cohen, F. L. (1980) Postsurgical pain relief: Patients' status and nurses' medication choices, *Pain*, 9:265–74.

Davitz, L. J. and Davitz, J. R. (1975) How nurses view patient suffering, *RN*, 38(10):69–72, 74.

Hackett, T. P. (1971) Pain and prejudice: Why do we doubt that the patient is in pain? *Medical Times*, 99(2):130–41.

Marks, R. M. and Sachar, E. J. (1973) Undertreatment of medical inpatients with narcotic analgesics, *Annals of Internal Medicine*, 78:173–81.

Osler, W. (1947) *The Hospital as a College*, Aequanimatas, The Blackstone Co.

Pilowsky, I. and Bond, M. R. (1969) Pain and its management in malignant disease, *Psychosomatic Medicine*, 31:400–4.

Seers, K. (1989) Patients' perception of acute pain, in *Directions in Nursing Research* (eds J. Wilson-Barnett and S. Robinson), pp. 107–16, Scutari Press.

Sofaer, B. (1984) *The Effect of Focused Education for Nursing Teams on Postoperative Pain of Patients*. Unpublished PhD thesis, University of Edinburgh.

Sternbach, R. A. (1968) *Pain: A Psychophysiological Analysis*, Academic Press.

Weis, O. F., Sriwatanakul, K., Alloza, J. L., Weintraub, M. and Lasagna, L. (1983) Attitudes of patients, housestaff and nurses towards postoperative analgesic care, *Anesthesia and Analgesia*, 62:72–4.

5

Accountability, responsibility, and communication

It sometimes seems that we are more concerned about minimizing patients' expression of pain than the pain itself.

(After McCaffery, 1983)

Accountability

Pain relief tends to be a low priority. For whatever reason – the lack of education or perhaps the organization of the system – members of health caring teams do not always hold themselves or each other accountable for relieving pain. Doctors write prescriptions. Nurses administer analgesics, but may not question in their own minds the efficacy or suitability of a medication for a particular patient, and may be reluctant to draw the attention of any shortcomings of the treatment to the doctor. If nurses do not involve themselves, the doctors' task will be made extremely difficult and sometimes impossible. One patient's comments illustrate the point of how sometimes analgesia is prescribed but not forthcoming when patients need it:

Once or twice I asked a nurse for tablets for the pain or for something to help me when I felt sick, but an hour or so later I was still waiting. Nobody ever came near me and I didn't know whether to ask them for anything again because nobody seemed to bother. You could ask a nurse something and she'd say, 'Right, I'll go and get sister' but nothing happened and you still weren't any better off. So half the time I thought there wasn't any point in asking them.

On the other hand, nurses often appear to control patients' *expression* of pain. A patient may be encouraged to 'Get hold of himself' or 'Not disturb other patients'. Sometimes a patient may feel uncomfortable about 'Bothering the nurse' because he has been told he can only have medication at certain times. This can be a particular problem at night when pain may keep him awake. It is not unknown for nurses to report that a patient had a 'good night' but for the patient to report that pain kept him awake.

It sometimes seems that we are more concerned about minimizing patients' expression of pain than the pain itself. Patients may sometimes be suffering in silence. The question of accountability for pain relief is therefore most important for nurses. Being accountable means realizing that we must share in a partnership with each patient. If a partnership exists, then the patient has a right to judge if the care is satisfactory. The pain is the *patient's* subjective experience.

Nurses must be able to offer the patient the opportunity to choose what may suit him best. This requires having a wide knowledge of coping strategies. More particularly, it requires attitudes on the part of nurses that allow patients to have control over their own pain and to maintain their self-respect. Patients should be encouraged not to feel that they must inevitably suffer pain. The way in which nursing care is organized may influence how nurses can exercise accountability. Where task allocation is practised, patients may come into contact with several nurses and the opportunity to develop a partnership in combating pain may not be there as much as when primary nursing is practised. However, nurses and patients are human and not everybody can achieve an excellent relationship. When a nurse finds herself in a situation such as this she should consult a colleague so that attempts can be made to help the patient.

Responsibility

Within certain limits, a nurse can choose how she moulds the situation in which she finds herself. She can either make active efforts to *change* situations and circumstances for the benefit of patients, or to remain ambivalent. For example, the nurse's interpretation of a prescription written four-hourly 'when necessary' can affect whether a patient suffers unnecessary pain or not. If the nurse interprets such a prescription to mean that she gives medication at the traditional drug round times only, she will deprive those patients whose requirements do not match her drug rounds. If, on the other hand, she assesses pain relief on an individual basis, patients are likely to benefit from pain *control* rather than pain *relief*, the implication here being that patients will be free from peaks of pain that occur as the effects of the drug wear off. Obviously, it takes time for each drug administration to have an effect, so patients could experience a considerable duration of pain if analgesia is only administered when pain becomes severe.

A further point is that nurses record that an analgesic drug or other pain relief measure has been administered but they seldom record the effect. Nurses should record and report pain in much more detail than is often done. If this were the case, then at the end of each shift the information collected would be helpful to the new shift of nurses in ensuring good continuity of care. It is also important to note how long it takes for a dose of medication to have an effect, how much relief it provides and how long the relief lasts. In addition, it is valuable to know how the medication was tolerated by the patient, and essential to know of any adverse effects. This information is not only of help to nurses but of inestimable value to the medical staff (Chapter 6).

Responsibility lies in the provision of human caring in general and the concerned provision of adequate pain control in particular. This should be based on a relationship between patient and nurse, which gives the patient 'space' to share in the decision-making. To achieve this requires skilled communication with nursing colleagues, patients, and doctors.

Communication

It is important to be aware that trust, respect, and empathy are essential to good communication. One reason why pain control may not be achieved is failure on the part of the nurse to realize that she has an important part to play. On the other hand, a nurse *may* realize the importance of her own rôle, but the process of communication with others may present difficulties. This might occur because of the organizational setting, or, as mentioned earlier, because a nurse brings certain of her own subjective experiences to the situation. In hospital settings, staff take for granted the day-to-day routines and this may blind them to some of the important aspects of interpersonal communication (Fagerhaugh and Strauss, 1977).

Some patients do not like to express their pain verbally. Others may find ways of distracting themselves, e.g. by knitting or watching television. Because they are occupied, they may not *appear* to be in pain, but we must not assume that pain is not present simply because their behaviour does not suggest that they are suffering.

Communication may be affected by the use of technical jargon and by health carers sometimes limiting themselves to giving information in a controlling way when communicating with patients in pain (Dangott *et al.*, 1978). One suggestion is that health carers should behave in a way that allows the patient to express himself in his own terms. For example, rather than *telling* the patient what a procedure may feel like, it would be more appropriate to allow him to express his *own* feelings in an atmosphere of openness, honesty and trust.

Figure 5.1 is a simple diagrammatic representation of communication between nurse, doctor, and a patient in pain. Figure 5.1(A) depicts

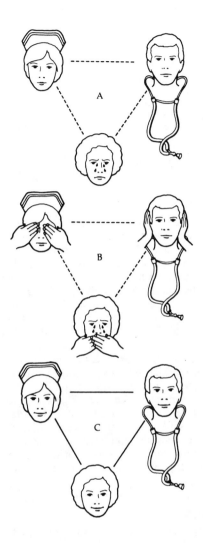

Figure 5.1 Diagramatic representations of communication between nurse, doctor, and a patient in pain. (A) potential communication; (B) non-communication; (C) successful communication. (Adapted from Sofaer (1987).)

potential communication, and is shown by broken lines. Figure 5.1(B) shows the patient not verbalizing her need for relief, the nurse 'not seeing' and the doctor 'not hearing'. In Figure 5.1(C), the patient is shown as pain-free and smiling, and the line of communication between the three people is unbroken.

Nurses and doctors

The interaction between nurses and doctors is of great importance in pain control. Sometimes relationships are less harmonious than they might be, and expectations of each other may be unrealistic. Doctors rely on nurses for reports, and nurses may be able to help the doctor to see the patient's point of view. Sometimes, however, nurses do not like to 'question' a doctor's 'judgement' of a situation; yet no doctor would wish a patient to suffer, and most welcome recognition by a nurse that analgesia is ineffective. The following anecdote (Sofaer, 1983b) illustrates a sad lack of communication:

A senior charge nurse complained that one of the anaesthetists had been prescribing the same amount of postoperative analgesia on a four-hourly 'as necessary' basis for 30 years. 'It's not a satisfactory arrangement', she said, 'Sometimes a patient requires the medication more frequently and at other times in an increased dose'. When asked why she could not simply request the doctor to be a little more flexible in his prescribing, or request a change of prescription by the houseman, she said, 'It's hospital policy that the anaesthetist writes up the postoperative medication for the first 24 hours' and 'We've been working together for 30 years and it's impossible to fight with him'.

It was suggested that she might try using a postoperative pain assessment chart [Chapter 6] and seeking the anaesthetist's assistance when analgesia was not effective. When the anaesthetist was told that the ward would be trying out an assessment chart, he said 'That's a good idea. I always prescribe four-hourly "as necessary" for the first 24 hours and I am always concerned that patients may suffer unnecessarily because the staff don't know how to interpret the prescription on the basis of individual needs. Nobody ever phones me! I've been working with the charge nurse for 30 years now and it would be quite impossible to tell her what to do.'

Even after 30 years of poor communication between two professional people, both of whom 'cared' in their own way, it was possible to improve postoperative pain management by making the recording of pain more systematic. In addition, a teaching programme was implemented on the ward, aimed at increasing knowledge and awareness of staff. This combined approach may have helped them towards increasing responsibility and accountability in this area (Sofaer, 1983a).

Nurses sometimes *blame* doctors – doctors sometimes *blame* nurses. It would be more helpful to find ways of communicating in an understanding way, recognizing that trust and respect are beneficial all round, especially to the patient. Twycross and Lack (1983) have also emphasized the importance of teamwork in the relief of pain, particularly in terminal care.

Keeping the patient informed

One aspect of communication often important for patients' peace of mind is the need for doctors and nurses to explain, in terms that a patient understands, the physiological or pathological basis for pain. Patients may sometimes have mistaken ideas of the pathological processes involved and these can be more terrifying than the actual disease. For example, I recently encountered two patients who were very concerned about their future bladder (urinary) function have undergone cholecystectomy. They thought that the gall bladder was part of the urinary system! Simple anatomical drawings or illustrations can obviously help to dispel such misconceptions. A brief summary of any explanation given can be written in the case notes and nursing care plan so that colleagues will be aware of what has been done and of any metaphor or analogy used.

Summary

- Pain relief tends to be a low priority.
- Nurses must assume accountability for providing pain relief.
- If a nurse assesses pain on an individual basis, then a patient is more likely to benefit from pain *control*.
- A record of both the administration and the effect of an analgesic would be helpful to a new shift of nurses coming on duty.
- Trust, respect, and empathy are essential to good communication.
- Good interaction between nursing and medical staff is important for patients' pain control.
- Appropriate explanations of the physiological or pathological basis of a patient's pain may contribute to his peace of mind.

References

Dangott, L., Thornton, B. C. and Page, P. (1978) Communication and pain, *Journal of Communication*, 28:30–5.

Fagerhaugh, S. Y. and Strauss, A. (1977) *Politics of Pain Management: Staff–patient Interaction*, Addison-Wesley Publishing Co.

McCaffery, M. (1983) *Nursing the Patient in Pain*, Harper & Row.

Sofaer, B. (1983a) The effect of focused nursing education on postoperative pain relief: a pilot study, in *Proceedings of the First Open Conference of the Workgroup for European Nurse Researchers*, Swedish Nurses Association.

Sofaer, B. (1983b) Pain relief: the importance of communication, *Nursing Times*, 79(48):32–5.

Sofaer, B. (1987) Pain. Helping to meet the challenge from a nursing point of view, in *Nursing the Physically Ill Adult* (eds J. R. P. Boore, R. Champion and M. C. Ferguson), Churchill Livingstone.

Twycross, R. G. and Lack, S. A. (1983) *Symptom Control in Far Advanced Cancer: Pain Relief*, Pitman Books Ltd.

6

Assessing pain

When we can assess the patient's pain accurately, we can treat it more effectively.

(McCaffery 1983)

Recognition of 'pain cues'

The process of pain assessment requires active effort on the part of the nurse and must begin with the recognition that pain is a subjective experience. In order to provide relief for a patient, the nurse must be able to recognize 'pain cues' and to evaluate the extent of the suffering. The task is not an easy one, and even very experienced nurses may underestimate the severity of a patient's pain.

One reason for the difficulty is that both patients and nurses have values and beliefs that vary on how one is expected to react to and report pain. For example, a nurse may expect a patient to show objective signs of pain. These may include elevated blood pressure, increased pulse and respiration rates, and perspiration. She may expect a patient to communicate his pain verbally, or she may expect a patient to show signs of pain through non-verbal behaviour such as writhing or restlessness.

However, although these cues may be present in some patients, lack of expressions of pain or lack of objective signs of pain does not necessarily mean lack of pain. Patients may adapt to pain both behaviourally and physiologically, perhaps because they place a high value on self-control, so that signs of suffering may be suppressed. Furthermore, because illness and pain are fatiguing, sometimes patients react by being quieter than usual and by lying still simply because they are too tired to do otherwise. It also could be that nurses expect others to control their feelings because they themselves have to do so in situations of stress (McCaffery, 1983).

Coping strategies of patients

Some patients may show minimal response to pain because they have devised their own coping strategies for distracting themselves. Under certain circumstances, nurses may not fully appreciate that a patient is watching television, knitting, or listening to music to take his mind off his pain. Often patients do not tell the staff about the methods they have devised to cope with pain, with the result that a decrease in pain expression may be misinterpreted by staff as meaning that pain has diminished or disappeared. For some patients, the expression of pain would make them feel ashamed or embarrassed.

Walker *et al.* (1990) have shown that for elderly patients suffering pain in the community personal strategies were important in maintaining control over chronic pain. Thus the assessment of patients' coping status could pave the way for more patient-centred care. Walker *et al.*'s assessment scheme for elderly patients is based on wide literature on pain and care of the elderly patient, but it is a scheme which could be utilized or adapted to meet the needs of many patients who suffer chronic pain (Figure 6.1).

Pain tolerance

Pain tolerance is the intensity of pain that an individual is willing to accept without seeking relief. Sometimes patients are referred to by staff as having a low pain tolerance. This may be disapproved of by some nursing staff who themselves value stoicism and admire people with willpower. This judgement may interfere with a nurse's assessment of pain and militate against effecting relief. A person's ability to tolerate pain may be affected by the psychological and cultural factors that have been discussed earlier, including anxiety level and past experiences. A fellow passenger on a train recalled to the author how he had suffered when having fluid aspirated from a very painful and swollen knee: 'It was outrageous. I never thought that pain could be so terrible. I had trusted the staff. They didn't offer me any pain-killers either before or afterwards. I will think twice before allowing doctors or nurses near me again.'

Nurses' acceptance of patients' statements

It may be that some patients do not spontaneously verbalize pain. When a patient does, it is important that the patient's report of pain is accepted. Very occasionally a nurse may care for a 'malingerer', but, generally speaking, side-effects of medication are unwanted and malingerers are few. Accepting and believing statements and reports of pain may rule out the possibility of a patient suffering unnecessarily.

Many people who suffer chronic pain learn to control the expression of their pain, and it would be a mistake not to believe such people on occasions when they report pain.

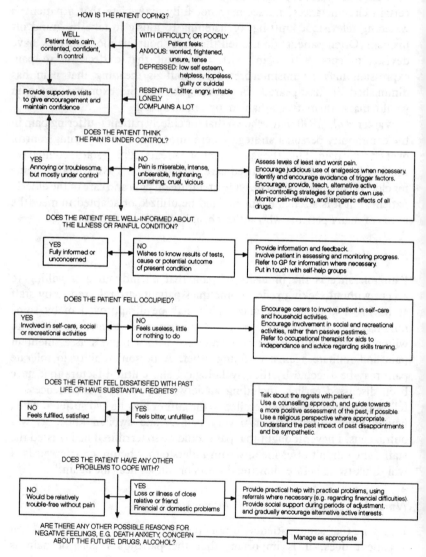

Figure 6.1 The nursing management of elderly patients with pain, in the community. From Walker, J. M., *et al.* (1990) The nursing management of elderly patients with pain in the community. *J. Advanced Nursing*, 15:1160, with permission.

Difficulties of assessing pain

In one study, nurses were asked to describe one patient situation in which it was difficult to assess pain and one in which it was easy. In general, nurses reported that physiological signs and behaviours were easier to note in assessing pain than verbal reports from the patient. Nurses did not rely so much on the patient's own reports of pain, even though the most reliable indicator of how much pain a person is experiencing is his own verbal subjective report (Jacox, 1979). However, this does not mean that subjective reports are the only ways of assessing pain. We must *begin* with the recognition that pain is a subjective phenomenon, and include the many factors influencing pain in our evaluation.

Misconceptions that may hamper the assessment of pain

The amount of tissue damage is not an accurate predictor of the intensity and duration of pain that a patient may suffer. Sometimes staff may think that patients undergoing similar surgical operations will experience the same intensity and/or duration of pain. The gate control theory of pain proposed by Melzack and Wall (1965) suggested that pain perception may be altered by cerebral influences. Past experiences, anxiety level, and the context of the trauma may therefore influence a person's response to pain.

The study of wounded soldiers in the Second World War referred to earlier (Chapter 2) showed that only 25% of badly injured men complained of pain or requested analgesia, whereas in a group of male civilians undergoing surgery, 80% required analgesia although their tissue damage was similar to that of the soldiers. The soldiers may have seen their wounds as a way of releasing them from duty at the front line and, because they sustained their injuries in a heroic context, they experienced less pain than the civilians who saw surgery as an interruption of their daily lives (Beecher, 1956). A more recent study of patients who underwent appendicectomy in Lebanon following the war in 1975–6 showed that these patients required less analgesia postoperatively than a similar group of patients who underwent similar surgery before the war. The findings implied that patients' perception of pain had changed due to the psychological trauma of war, resulting in patients requiring less analgesia to relieve postoperative pain (Armenian *et al.*, 1981).

Routine and tradition

Assessment of pain is further hampered by 'routine' drug rounds in hospitals and/or caring institutions. This routine places constraints on patients who may feel they have to ask for analgesics at that time, or accept them if offered. This may be done simply to comply with the ward routine or because a patient knows that the trolley may not be round for another four hours and that he could experience pain before then but not want to bother a nurse. One patient mentioned that she missed the six pm trolley because she went to the bathroom. She said, 'I was in agony – I thought the nurses would come back and ask me if I needed pain-killers, but they didn't. I think they must have been very busy and I didn't like to ask, so I waited for the night nurses' drug round.'

Should patients be expected to gear their pain relief requirements to hospital routines? Good assessment of a patient's pain may reveal that this requirement is either more or less than that which is made available to him from the four-hourly drug trolley round.

Awareness of pain should be a routine item in caring for patients. Edwards (1990) defines the problem of undertreatment of patients as originating in deficiencies in knowledge and skills of staff. In a study to test the effect of education for nurses on postoperative pain of patients, Sofaer (1984) found that greater proportions of patients felt their pain was noticed by staff after the educational programme for staff. The programme highlighted the importance of assessment.

Individualized assessment of pain

One argument that has been offered by nurses against individualized assessment of pain is that medical staff often prescribe analgesia 'four-hourly' (which may be true even though duration of action of an analgesic is less than four hours). This does not mean that the nurse must interpret the time of administration necessarily to coincide with routine drug rounds. The whole point of pain assessment is that it will reveal whether or not the prescriptional framework within which a drug is administered is appropriate for an individual patient. If not, the medical staff can be approached and asked if they would be willing to alter the prescription, either to increase or decrease a dose or to increase or decrease the frequency of administration, or to prescribe an alternative analgesic with a different intensity or duration of action. One staff nurse using pain assessment commented, 'Each patient's assessments show a different pattern and their individual requirements vary.'

It is worth mentioning that in the case of morphine the reason for prescribing it four hourly is to avoid cumulative effects. If you give morphine three hourly, it cumulates as seen in Figure 6.2. Whereas when given four hourly, the level in the blood has time to return to normal base level, as seen in Figure 6.3. However, the base level *must* be high enough, and that is achieved by giving a big enough dose. So, if a drug is wearing off before the four hours is up, the doctor should be approached with a view to increasing the dose. This can be seen by careful assessment by the nurse. If morphine is only going to be given for a 24-hour period, then cumulation is not a hazard, but if it is given over two to three days, it is.

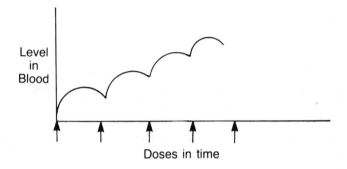

Figure 6.2

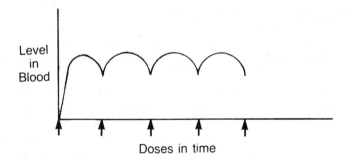

Figure 6.3

The responsibility of the nurse

Because of the individual nature of pain and the variation in its expression, nurses must be prepared to accept some of the responsibility in identifying when a patient is in pain. One way of trying to overcome the difficulties is to use a pain assessment chart (Figure 6.4).

The main advantage of having a written record of pain assessment is that it improves the chance of decreasing suffering by facilitating communication between patients, nurses, and medical staff. In one ward where pain assessment had been recorded as part of a research project on the management of postoperative pain, a staff nurse said, 'I feel much more in control of the situation now than before. I am less anxious myself about the possibility of patients suffering unnecessarily. The assessment chart is easy to use and has helped us all to control pain before it gets severe.'

Learning what a patient is experiencing

In order to be effective in her intervention, the nurse must not only be observant, she must be able to examine the factors influencing the patient's pain response and minimize her own prejudices about how pain should be tolerated. There is also the need to find out how the patient usually deals with pain, and to enlist his assistance in assessing the pain and in finding ways to relieve it. Above all, a nurse must always be willing to listen to a patient in an empathetic way, and to accept that only the patient can really know what hurts, when it hurts and how much it hurts.

Assessing the pain with the patient

Pain is assessed *with* the patient and not *on* the patient. This is a very important point because the patient's own estimate of pain must be used as the basis for treatment. The nurse should not allow her own experiences of pain, or her observations in other situations, to influence the assessment.

Figure 6.4 illustrates a pain assessment chart showing how one patient's pain was assessed and relieved effectively following surgery. Figure 6.5 illustrates a chart showing how moderate pain was delayed, even though the nurse making the assessment informed the medical staff that analgesia was not effective. This patient experienced considerable suffering.

Protracted or chronic pain

In assessing protracted or chronic pain, a body chart may be helpful to the patient in locating pain. It also provides a means whereby the site of pain can be documented. You can make up a body chart by drawing a simple outline of the front and back views of the body. A patient may then be asked to indicate the site of his pain by marking the chart. Any changes can be noted on subsequent charts and recordings may be made

Sheet No. 1

PAIN ASSESSMENT CHART

Ward Z 8

Patient's Name: Mrs MacDonald

Hospital Number: 00 7413

Put a tick in the column which best describes the pain since the last recording

Date	Time	No pain or sleeping	Slight pain	Moderate pain	Severe pain	Pain bad as it could be	Signature of nurse	Site	Comment and/or nursing action	Analgesic given: Name	Dose	Route	Time
13·6·92	11 00		✓				P Smith	abdomen	analgesic given with anti emetic	Diamorphine	5mg.	I.M.	11 00
	12·10			✓			P Smith	abdomen	Discussed with Dr. analgesic given	Diamorphine	5mg	I.M.	12·15
	13·30	✓					P. Smith	–					
	14·30	✓					P. Smith	–					
	15·30			✓			S/N McCallum	abdomen	Analgesic and Antiemetic given	Omnopon	15 mg	I.M.	15·35
	16·30	✓					S/N McCallum	–	appears more settled				
	18·00	✓					S/N McCallum	–					
	20·00			✓			S/N Ford	abdomen	washed and turned mod. pain following ∴ analgesic given	Omnopon	15 mg	I.M.	20·10
	22·00	✓					S/N Ford	–	Turned and settled down.				
	24·00	✓					S/N T Burns	–					
14·6·92	01·45		✓				S/N T Burns	abdomen	Analgesic given	Omnopon	15 mg	I.M.	01·45

Figure 6.4 A pain-assessment chart showing how one patient's pain was assessed and effectively relieved following surgery.

Sheet No. 1

PAIN ASSESSMENT CHART

Ward B.

Patient's Name: Mrs Fraser.

Hospital Number: 274306.

Put a tick in the column which best describes the pain since the last recording

Date	Time	No pain or sleeping	Slight pain	Moderate pain	Severe pain	Pain bad as it could be	Signature of nurse	Site	Comment and/or nursing action	Analgesic given: Name	Dose	Route	Time
23·8·92	16·45				✓		P. Jones.	abdomen	Requested Dr. to increase dose (refused)	Diamorphine	2·5mg	I/M	17·10
	17·40			✓			P. Jones.	abdomen					
	19·10		✓				P. Jones.	abdomen					
	20·20	✓					P. Jones						
	21·15			✓			P. Jones.	abdomen	Requested Dr. to increase dose (refused)	Diamorphine	2·5mg	I/M	21·20
	22.00			✓			J. Frost.	abdomen					
	23·20			✓			J. Frost.	abdomen	Analgesia	Diamorphine	2·5mg	I/M	23·25
24·8·92	24·00	✓					J. Frost.						
	02·00		✓				M. Freeman	abdomen					
	03·30	✓					M. Freeman						
	04·00						M. Freeman	abdomen	Analgesic given	Diamorphine	2·5	I/M	04·00
	04·30	✓					M. Freeman						
	06·00	✓					M. Freeman						

Figure 6.5 A pain-assessment chart showing how pain relief was delayed.

of any action taken to relieve the pain. To elicit descriptions of pain and to assess changes in the nature and severity of pain over time, a pain description chart might be helpful. Patients may be asked to select from a list of adjectives such as 'mild', 'distressing', 'knifelike', 'throbbing' or 'cramping', those words that best describe the pain. It might also be possible to connect an episode of pain with a bodily function or a time of day and thereby help the patient to find ways of avoiding such pain-inducing situations.

Pain in children

Assessing pain in children may present further difficulties. The effectiveness of relevant play in preparing children for painful procedures is very important, but words are not reliable in communicating with very young children when trying to assess the location and intensity of pain. Play presents information in a more understandable way, and young children readily identify with and project feelings onto a special doll or teddy. A nurse could therefore exploit such play to find out the location of pain using the doll or teddy. An older child might be able to point to the site of pain on a body chart. (For an excellent text on pain and children see McGrath and Unruh, 1987.)

Use of an analogue scale

Since pain is a subjective experience, it may be useful to provide a patient with a scale on which the extremes of the experience are indicated (Figure 6.6).

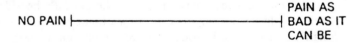

Figure 6.6 A visual analogue scale (after Scott and Huskisson, 1976).

The patient is asked to place a mark on the scale to represent the level of pain at the time. The distance of the mark from the left-hand end of the scale is the pain score. The scale may be used several times during a day. A pain profile (Figure 6.7) may then be constructed to show if treatment has been effective.

Intervals between pain assessments

There are no set rules regarding the time interval between pain assessments for the same patient. It is, however, important that nurses

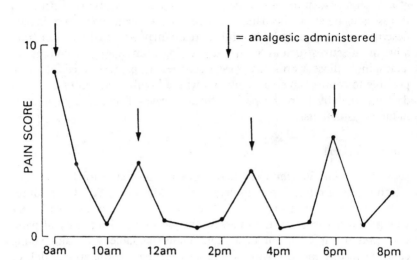

Figure 6.7 A pain profile showing the effect of analgesia on pain score (after Bond, 1979). Arrows indicate the times at which an analgesic was administered.

record the administration and subsequent effect of an analgesic or other pain-relieving strategy. Circumstances vary from one situation to another. It may be that following surgery pain assessment would be appropriate every two or three hours for the first two to three days, with the frequency of assessment being decreased subsequently. It is strongly recommended that the assessment chart is left at the patient's bedside. Since no patient would be left for more than two hours without some member of staff coming to the bedside, the process of pain assessment does not involve extra staff and requires little additional time.

Patients who experience chronic pain might find it helpful to have their pain assessed twice daily to check the efficacy of analgesia. For patients who are nursed at home, a home assessment record could be useful in disclosing patterns of pain and facilitating adjustments in therapy by the doctor.

Comfort measures

Re-positioning, smoothing the bed, and offering a warm drink can help a patient to relax. Although these measures may not relieve severe pain, they may sometimes relieve discomfort or mild pain, making more potent therapies unnecessary. The following anecdote illustrates this point. A patient returned from the operating theatre following a trans-urethral prostatectomy. He reported pain, and an opioid analgesic was administered. The cause of the pain was not investigated. He remained restless and agitated and looked unwell. The staff nurse noticed that the urethral catheter was not draining, so she performed a bladder washout. A litre of fluid was removed. The patient settled, slept well, and his colour returned to normal. The nurse later commented that in this instance an obvious cause for the pain had been a full bladder, and that it had served as a good learning experience, where an analgesic had not been required and should not have been given prior to other measures being taken.

Patients' views

The experience of pain has been described by one author as including both the stimulus and response to that stimulus, and she has analyzed the 'experience' of patients in terms of 'suffering' (Copp, 1974). In the course of her research she asked patients what nurses and doctors could do about pain. Patients suggested that there is nothing more important than talking to patients about pain and that nurses should be prompt and try to understand. Nurses should also stop telling people they do not have pain when they actually do and not try to feel *for* people when they can't know if patients have pain or not. Having confidence can help relieve the pain – if nurses had more confidence patients would too. Patients also felt that nurses should not assume that medication helps. In addition, Copp examined how nurses appear to patients in response to a request for pain relief. A patient may see the nurse as acting in a variety of roles, e.g. one of the following:

- A *controller* – relieving or denying relief.
- A *communicator* – passing on, validating, and interpreting the bid for pain reduction.
- A *judge* – deciding if pain is reasonable, timely, and expected in terms of quality and quantity.
- An *avoider* – refusing to report that medication does not bring relief.
- An *empathizer* – letting the patient have his own experience; an authentic empathizer 'knows' and 'has experiences'; a pseudo-empathizer responds by describing her own experience to obtain feelings of credit, or to rob the patient of attention.
- A *barterer* – giving relief in return for good patient behaviour.

An awareness by nurses of how their own behaviour might affect a patient's response to pain and its assessment have further implications. For example, if a nurse acts in a judgemental way, relief may be given to the patient in order to salve the nurse's conscience and not because the nurse herself really believes in what the patient is saying.

Prerequisites for nurses assessing pain

A background knowledge of the theoretical concepts involved in the complex phenomenon of pain is the first step. Displaying acceptance of individual patient's differences in pain tolerance and coping patterns are also basic prerequisites for any nurse who wishes to be effective in relieving pain.

Summary

- Pain assessment requires active effort on the part of the nurse.
- Patients have individual coping strategies.
- It is important that nurses accept patients' statements about pain.
- There are some misconceptions which may hamper assessment of pain.
- Ward routines place constraints on patients' requests for pain relief.
- Pain assessment may help to reveal whether or not a particular drug is appropriate for a patient.
- A pain assessment chart provides a written record and facilitates communication between patients, nurses, and doctors.
- In assessing pain with children, play may help in finding out the location of pain.
- Although there are no set rules for timing of pain assessment, nurses should record the administration and effect of each pain-relieving strategy.
- Patients have several suggestions about what nurses and doctors can do about pain.
- Patients may see nurses as acting in one of a variety of roles in response to patients' pain.
- A background knowledge about pain is a first step to assessing pain with patients.

References

Armenian, H. K., Chamieh, M. A. and Barak, A. (1981) Influences of war-time stress and psychosocial factors in Lebanon on analgesic requirements for post-operative pain, *Social Science and Medicine*, 151:63–6.

Beecher, H. K. (1956) Relationship of significance of wound to pain experienced, *Journal of the American Medical Association*, 161:1609–13.

Bond, M. R. (1979) *Pain: Its Nature, Analysis and Treatment*, Churchill Livingstone.

Copp, L. A. (1974) The spectrum of suffering, *American Journal of Nursing*, 74:491–5.

Edwards, W. T. (1990) Optimizing opioid treatment of postoperative pain. *Journal of Pain and Symptom Management*, 5 Feb (1 Supp), S24–36.

Jacox, A. K. (1979) Assessing pain, *American Journal of Nursing*, 79:895–900.

McCaffery, M. (1983) *Nursing the Patient in Pain*, Harper & Row.

McGrath, P. J. and Unruh, A. M. (1987) *Pain in Children and Adolescents*.

Melzack, R. and Wall, P. D. (1965) Pain mechanisms: A new theory, *Science*, 150:971–9.

Scott, J. and Huskisson, E. C. (1976) Graphic representation of pain, *Pain*, 2:175–84.

Sofaer, B. (1984) *The Effect of Focused Education for Nursing Teams on Postoperative Pain of Patients*. Unpublished PhD thesis, University of Edinburgh.

Walker, J. M., Akinsanya, J. A., Davis, B. D. and Marcer, D. (1989) The nursing management of elderly patients with pain in the community: study and recommendations. *Journal of Advanced Nursing*, 15:1154–61.

7

Pain therapies

We have learned as a result of literally hundreds of experiments, that there is a limit to the effectiveness of any given therapy; but happily the effects of two or more therapies given in combination are cumulative.

(Melzack and Wall 1982)

So far this book has focused on the complex nature of pain. The traditional approach to treating pain has been to use invasive methods; that is to say, methods that physically invade or enter the body. Examples of these methods are analgesics, nerve blocks, or surgical procedures. Increasingly, however, it is being recognized that, because so many factors influence the nature of pain, both the local tissue damage and innumerable external factors, it is best to treat pain (acute or chronic) using a combined physical and psychological approach.

The therapies outlined below could easily be used in such an integrated way. Some of them lie directly within the province of the nurse; for example, distraction techniques, guided imagery, and relaxation are all non-invasive methods that nurses can initiate without a doctor's prescription. If a particular method does not work it can be discarded. The nurse should try to individualize each method to suit a particular patient and his pain. Sometimes patients can be taught to use these techniques on their own. There is some degree of overlap between the different methods.

Nurses do not, however, prescribe medications, although they do have considerable 'power' in relation to the administration of analgesics. In this respect, nurses must be familiar particularly with the rules regarding administration and the possible side-effects. Nurses also do not carry out local anaesthetic blocks, but do have a role here in preparing and supporting patients before and during this treatment.

Distraction

Distraction is when someone focuses attention on a stimulus other than the pain. Sometimes distraction can or has to be used without planning or explanation. On other occasions, a nurse may plan beforehand and rehearse with a patient a particularly useful strategy prior to a painful procedure. It may be helpful to boost the confidence of the patient by taking an opportunity to practice while he is pain-free. The quality of the nurse–patient relationship will influence the patient's willingness to try a particular technique.

Some patients use distraction themselves, without being taught, but do not tell the staff that they are consciously doing so. Reading, listening to music, or watching television are examples of distraction. Imagination (mental imagery) is another form of distraction. Distraction may increase a patient's tolerance for pain and sometimes decrease the intensity of pain. What seems to happen is that pain ceases to be the focus of the patient's attention.

Unfortunately, many health professionals doubt that a patient is in pain if he is able to distract himself or be distracted (Wiener, 1975). One comment overheard from a nurse was that a patient was 'sitting up in bed chatting happily to visitors', the assumption being that the patient could not possibly have been experiencing much pain. Perhaps the patient was being distracted from his pain. In one study it was found that patients developed their own coping behaviours at home but felt that doctors or nurses 'might not like it'. They felt that their coping behaviours might be 'against the rules' and might be laughed at as not being scientific (Copp, 1974).

Following the use of distraction, increased awareness of pain and fatigue may be present. A patient should, therefore, be provided with an appropriate alternative method of relief following distraction. Another approach is to use distraction consciously while waiting for other methods to take effect. One patient said, 'I listen to music while waiting for the pain-killers to take effect.'

Distraction alone is a potent pain reliever in certain situations. For example, when changing dressings, nurses can distract patients by getting them to talk about a favourite pastime, a book they may be reading, or their family. If patients do not feel like talking, another useful strategy is one described by McCaffery (1983). The nurse suggests to the patient that he stares at a spot (anything close at hand, from a flower to a door knob) during which an area of skin is massaged in a slow, rhythmic, often circular, manner. The nurse can do this or the patient can do it for himself. The massage can be done on, or near, the painful area or on another part of the body depending on the nature of the injury or painful area. Another distraction strategy involves slow, rhythmic breathing (for use of this and pant–blow rhythmic breathing the reader is referred to McCaffery, 1983, pp. 151–5).

A method of distraction frequently used with children is to read stories to them and get them to describe the pictures. Adult patients can use pictures in a similar way, not only by looking at pictures of particular interest, but by using their senses in an imaginary way. For example, in looking at a picture of a country scene, the patient could imagine he hears the birds singing, feels the warmth of the sun on his skin and smells the fragrant flowers. This is using imagery in conjunction with distraction.

Imagery

The technique of imagery is different insofar as distraction is usually dependent on external stimuli, whereas imagery depends on the mind exclusively, usually through evoking visual sensations, although best results may be obtained by using all the senses. Imagery may be taught to a patient for distraction purposes. It may be preceded by a relaxation technique (page 62). Imagery, as taught to a patient for self use, gives the patient control over whether he will use it and when. In using imagery the patient is alert and concentrating very hard.

One example of the power of imagery is to imagine yourself slicing a lemon and arranging it on a dish. When did your mouth begin to water? Imagination seems to involve responses from both mind and body.

Progressive relaxation exercises, followed by imagining idyllic scenes, may be useful in relieving both acute and chronic pain. One person who tried imagery was a colleague with a severe migraine. Until he was able to get to a chemist shop and purchase medication, he tried the following technique. He imagined himself near a beach – he did not like the sun so he chose the shade of a tree in which to rest. When asked what he heard, smelled and felt, he replied that he heard the sound of the waves and of children playing, smelled the sea air and felt the breeze on his face. This imagery took about 15 minutes, by which time he had reached the chemist shop. It is useful to find out from a patient to what extent he already uses imagery as a pain-relieving technique, and it should be pointed out that imagery can be used along with other pain-relieving techniques.

If you guide the imagery you can use persuasive suggestions. For instance, you could say, 'When you are ready', or 'Perhaps you feel' (for example, the warmth of the sun). This approach involves the patient in deciding what is best for him. Sometimes people feel drowsy afterwards.

If the patient wants to sleep he can say to himself, 'When I awake I will feel fresh.' If he does not want to sleep, he could suggest to himself that when he has finished his imagining he will feel alert and awake.

Imagery can be used either for very brief periods or for a longer time, perhaps up to 20 minutes. One way to encourage a patient to use imagery is for the nurse to suggest to the patient that he pictures himself in a pleasant environment, for example in a park. The nurse can then ask the patient for a description of his surroundings, encouraging responses that use all his senses. If the patient has difficulty, the nurse could help by introducing appropriate images. For example, for one patient who was feeling very hot, it was suggested that she imagine herself resting under the shade of a big, leafy tree, feeling the cool breeze. Visual imagery can also be very helpful during uncomfortable procedures such as removal of sutures.

One specific image for pain relief involves picturing the pain flowing away from the body. McCaffery (1983, p. 262) describes instructions she gives to a patient with a tension headache. For patients with pain in another site, the word 'head' can be substituted with the appropriate site:

> Get into a comfortable position. Close your eyes now. Take a slow, rather deep breath, and feel yourself relax as you breathe out. Continue to breathe comfortably and slowly, feeling your body relax each time you breathe out. If you wish, the next time you breathe in you can imagine that your breath goes to your head, bringing nutrients, comfort and calm. As you breathe out, you can imagine that the air goes out through your head, taking with it the discomfort, leaving behind relaxed, healthy, comfortable tissues. Each time you breathe in you can picture the air flowing through to your head, bringing health and comfort. As you breathe out, the air once again flows out through your head, leaving calm, relaxation, health and comfort behind. I will pause now and you can continue to breathe slowly and imagine more and more comfort with each breath that flows through your head [Pause for whatever amount of time seems reasonable, for example, 15 s or 1 min.] When you are ready, you may end this image by counting silently to yourself from one to three. At the count of three inhale, open your eyes, and say to yourself that you feel alert and relaxed. I will wait now until you are ready to end this for yourself. Take your time. Enjoy the experience.

One variation is for the patient to imagine he is sitting on a river bank and with each breath out his pain flows down the river and out to sea.

Another image that may be useful is for the patient to imagine himself as healthy. The nurse can suggest to the patient the following short image as described by McCaffery (1983, p. 265):

> If you wish, you may begin to picture yourself as being healthy. Perhaps you would like to begin with your toes and slowly work upwards. You may find this easier to do with your eyes closed. You may see each part of your body forming just as you want it to be. You can paint this picture of yourself in your mind's eye or you can simply allow the picture to form

slowly. You can see that each body part is healthy. See yourself exactly as you want to be. See yourself healed. See each part of yourself functioning normally, inside and outside your body.

Using imagery with children can be particularly helpful. It could be the 'let's pretend' game. Allowing the child to imagine being his favourite hero in a story may be an acceptable way of helping him to cope with pain.

The use of colour, either in the environment or imagination, may be a useful aid. One patient used six coloured bangles as an aid to help her imagine the sun, sea and earth, and was able to create some very beautiful images for herself.

Relaxation exercises used in conjunction with imagery may enhance the effect of the imagery.

Relaxation techniques

Relaxation is freedom from mental and physical tension and stress. There are several techniques available to achieve a state of relaxation, all requiring the patient's participation. One or more techniques may often be combined with other therapies such as counselling to make a programme that may sometimes be referred to as relaxation therapy. What are described here are individual techniques. As mentioned earlier, any of these may also be used prior to using imagery to enhance its effect.

Many patients already practise some form of a relaxation technique. The nurse should enquire about this and if a patient finds a particular technique helpful, the nurse should encourage its use.

Relaxation may be achieved by various means, for example meditation, yoga or progressive relaxation exercises. Whatever technique is used, the aim should be to reduce the effect of stress. It is not clear how stress and pain are related but it may be that stress aggravates pain. It is, however, generally recognized that there is a relationship between pain and tension and anxiety. Relaxation techniques may also help to lower anxiety. This may, in certain circumstances, be helpful to overanxious patients. A further point is that a relaxation technique can act as a distraction so that the patient's mind is taken off the pain. Muscle relaxation training has been found to decrease 'state anxiety', that is anxiety which may be present in patients facing potentially stressful events (Johnson and Spielberger, 1968). Relaxation may help a patient to sleep. Since pain is fatiguing it is a useful strategy in overcoming fatigue.

Some people have erroneous beliefs that relaxing is achieved by reading a book or watching television. In these situations, a person may still feel stressed. It is important to realize that people need to *learn* relaxation techniques. It is helpful if one can choose a quiet environment and assume a comfortable position to practice relaxation. Some people like to lie down, others prefer to sit in a straight-backed chair.

A technique recommended by McCaffery (1983, p. 221), which can be accomplished quickly, is to:

1. Breathe in deeply and clench your fists.
2. Breathe out and go limp as a rag doll.
3. Start yawning.

Repeat these instructions as often as necessary. Step 1 should always be followed by Step 2, but Steps 2 and 3 can be repeated alone at intervals.

Slow, rhythmic breathing can also be effective. It is often helpful for patients who experience chronic pain and who may like to use some method of relaxation regularly. The nurse can teach the patient to do abdominal breathing, and then instruct them as follows (McCaffery, 1983, p. 223):

1. Close your eyes and take a slow, deep breath.
2. As you breathe out, feel yourself relax. Feel the tension draining out of your body.
3. Breathe slowly and comfortably from your abdomen.
4. Think about your breathing. Feel the air enter your nose and lungs. Feel the air go out of your lungs, and feel yourself relaxing as you breathe out.
5. To help you breathe slowly and rhythmically, as you inhale I will say 'in, one two'; as you exhale, 'out, one, two'. (Say these phrases in co-ordination with the patient's breathing in and out. Do this two or three times to help the patient slow his breathing and keep it regular.)
6. Feel yourself relax each time you breathe out. Just let the air flow from your lungs and let the tension flow from your body.
7. As you breathe in you may say silently to yourself, 'In, one, two'. As you breathe out you may say to yourself, 'Relax'. (Say these phrases two or three times in co-ordination with the patient's breathing. A word other than 'relax' may have been chosen by the patient prior to using the technique.)
8. I am going to pause now to let you concentrate on your breathing. Relax as you breathe out, breathing slowly and rhythmically, counting silently for yourself if you wish. (Watch the patient, and if tension or difficulty arises, begin the counting for him and repeat the instructions in step 7.)

9. When you are ready to end this relaxation you may do so yourself.
When you are ready, count silently from one to three. At the count of
three, inhale deeply, silently say to yourself, 'I feel alert and relaxed',
and open your eyes. I will wait now for you to end your relaxation for
yourself when you are ready.

It may be helpful for some patients if the nurse puts the instructions on
tape, possibly including some guided imagery. For home-care patients
this may be particularly useful since they could play the tape whenever
they felt the need. A useful adjunct is an earpiece so as not to disturb
other patients or, if at home, members of a family.

Some problems may occasionally arise. For example, a person may
become very aware of body sensations or become withdrawn. Alternatively, patients may complain that techniques are 'boring'. Perhaps
modifying the technique would help. If not, the nurse should discuss
with the patient the possibility of discontinuing its use.

Analgesics

The administration of analgesic drugs is a common method of pain relief.
Because doctors prescribe the drugs, it is sometimes assumed that
understanding them is solely a medical responsibility. However, it is
particularly important that nurses, too, understand how analgesics work
since it is to nurses that patients will often turn for pain relief. Control of
pain often depends on nursing staff, for nurses hold the keys of the
cupboard where analgesics are kept. It is nurses who can exercise their
discretion so that patients have the maximum control of pain. Too often
the power that nurses have in this respect is used negatively, without
individual assessment of pain and without any knowledge of drug
potency.

In discussing potency, a distinction is drawn between opioid analgesics
and non-opioid analgesics. Opioid analgesics work by acting on the
central nervous system, whereas non-opioid analgesics act on the nerves
at the site of pain. Opioid analgesics such as morphine are usually the
only effective drugs in combatting severe pain, whereas non-opioid
analgesics such as aspirin are helpful for relief of mild to moderate pain.
Opioid analgesics are not useful in pain which is not responsive to
opioids, such as bone pain.

The ideal analgesic drug should be easily administered, effective, safe,
and cheap. The most important criterion is safety, but as with all drugs,
the use of both opioids and non-opioids carries risks. Some commonly

used opioid and non-opioid analgesic drugs are described below, but this is by no means a comprehensive list and is only intended as an introduction to the subject. Latham (1990) has summarized the use of drugs in pain control, and for even more advanced information the reader is advised to consult a clinical pharmacology text.

Opioid analgesia

Opioid analgesics affect perception of pain by acting on the central nervous system. They are used to relieve severe pain and also may produce a sense of well-being. This is linked with the tendency of these drugs sometimes to produce mental and physical dependence. Opioids include both natural and synthetic drugs and are also known as opiates or morphine and its congeners. Opioid analgesics are subject to the provisions of the Misuse of Drugs Act, 1971 and have to be prescribed by a medical or dental practitioner. They are therefore called controlled drugs.

The 1985 Misuse of Drugs Regulations has specified the classes of people who are authorized to supply and possess controlled drugs in their capacity as professionals. Drugs are controlled depending on their formulation. Five schedules are identified in the regulations. Schedules two and three particularly apply to analgesics. Schedule two drugs are those which are subject to full control. They have to be prescribed in writing, have to be in safe custody, and they have to be recorded in registers. Examples include morphine, diamorphine, pethidine, and injectable pentazocine. Schedule three drugs require a special prescription but are not subject to safe custody or register requirements. A requirement is that invoices have to be kept for two years. Drugs which come under these regulations include buprenorphine and oral pentazocine.

There are two types of regulation regarding administration of drugs: first, Statutory Regulations relating to Acts of Parliament, and, second, local hospital regulations. Individual Health Authorities also draw up guidelines for storage and administration of medicines. Doses referred to below are adult doses given in the British National Formulary (1990).

Morphine The most commonly used opioid analgesic is morphine, a derivative of opium. The usual dose for an adult is 10–20 mg administered intramuscularly or subcutaneously. The duration of action of morphine is usually considered to be about four hours, but this should not be taken for granted because of individual variation. Pain relief following administration should be assessed according to the guidelines in Chapter 6. The major side-effect of morphine is dose-related respiratory depression. Care is needed in situations where this could be dangerous, e.g. in patients with pulmonary disease. Overdose of morphine can suppress respiration completely and cause death. The depressant effect of morphine on the respiratory system can be counteracted by administering a specific morphine antagonist. The drug of choice for reversing the effect of morphine is naloxone.

Other side effects of morphine may be nausea and/or vomiting with the initial doses. Usually, therefore, an anti-emetic drug is prescribed with morphine. Morphine can also be administered orally and is suitable for relief of pain in terminal care. A simple elixir of morphine and water may be prescribed together with an anti-emetic such as prochlorperazine. A dose of 20–30 mg of morphine in an oral solution is generally considered to be equivalent to 10 mg of morphine by injection. Morphine can also be administered by rectum using suppositories. These come in 15 mg and 30 mg strengths. A sustained-release form of morphine is available in tablet form (MST Continus, 10 mg, 30 mg, 60 mg and 100 mg strengths). This is a long-acting preparation which may be helpful in domiciliary care for the relief of prolonged and severe pain. The dose is dependent on the severity of the pain. MST Continus may also be used for the relief of postoperative pain.

Morphine induces constriction of the pupils of the eyes. It also decreases peristaltic activity of the gastrointestinal tract. One side-effect of this is constipation. Constipation is inevitable with the use of opioids, and patients need strong stimulant laxatives. If someone is going to be given opioids for more than 24 hours, they should be given laxatives routinely. Further possible side-effects are lowering of the blood pressure, dizziness, and itching of the skin. One feature of morphine therapy is the development of patient tolerance; that is, the need to administer increasingly large doses to produce the same analgesic effect. If clinical tolerance develops, it is important to realize that this cannot be equated with addiction. There is also no reason to believe that it will lead to addiction (Jaffe, 1975). Drug abuse is a voluntary behaviour. Drug tolerance and physical dependence are involuntary behaviours based on physiological changes that take place within the body.

Diamorphine (heroin) Diamorphine is a derivative of morphine. Following administration, the effect of diamorphine has a more rapid onset and shorter duration than that of morphine. The usual dose is 5–10 mg, given intramuscularly or subcutaneously. Diamorphine can also be given in oral solution, 13–20 mg given orally being equivalent to 4–5 mg by injection. Diamorphine causes greater respiratory depression than morphine.

Papaveretum (Omnopon) Papaveretum is given to relieve moderate to severe pain. It does not appear to have any advantage over morphine. It consists of 50% morphine and 50% other opium alkaloids. A dose of 13.5 mg of papaveretum is equal to 10 mg of morphine sulphate. It can be given by injection, subcutaneously, intramuscularly, or intravenously (10–20 mg) and is also available in 10 mg tablets.

Pethidine This is a synthetic drug unrelated to morphine. It is a powerful analgesic that also reduces muscle spasm. It is very useful for the treatment of renal and biliary colic, and labour pain. The usual dose is 50–100 mg given intramuscularly. Following administration, the onset of its effect is rapid, but duration of action tends to be shorter than morphine, usually about two to three hours. Again, nurses should regularly assess the efficacy of the drug *with* individual patients to avoid unnecessary pain. Medical staff should be informed if the prescription provided does not allow for administration within the time that the patient experiences renewed pain. There may be less respiratory depression than with morphine, but pethidine should not be given to patients who are taking psychotropic drugs of the monoamine oxidase inhibitor group as excitation, coma, changes in blood pressure or death could occur. As with morphine, tolerance and dependence can develop.

Dihydrocodeine tartrate (DF118) Dihydrocodeine tartrate (DF118) is administered orally (30–60 mg) or intramuscularly (50 mg). If given intramuscularly it is regarded as a controlled drug, if given orally it is not. It is used for the relief of moderate to severe pain. Side effects are dizziness, nausea and constipation.

Codeine phosphate Codeine phosphate is administered orally (10–60 mg) or intramuscularly (up to 30 mg). Tolerance and dependence are common. Side effects are dizziness, nausea, and constipation.

Phenazocine (Narphen) This analgesic is effective for severe pain, particularly biliary colic. Nausea and vomiting may occur, and if so the drug can be administered sublingually. The oral dose is 5–20 mg.

Methadone (Physeptone) Methadone may be administered for severe pain. It is less effective and sedating than morphine. It is sometimes used for the relief of terminal pain. The injections may cause local pain and tissue damage. The usual dose is 5–10 mg which can be administered subcutaneously or intramuscularly. By mouth the dose is usually 20 mg. Methadone may have a greater respiratory depressant effect than morphine. In some situations it is used to suppress intractable cough and dyspnoea.

Buprenorphine (Temgesic)   Buprenorphine is used to treat moderate to severe pain. The side-effects are less marked than those of morphine, although it may be helpful to give an anti-emetic over the first few days of administration. The effects of buprenorphine may not be reversed by naloxone. It may therefore antagonize analgesia from large doses of morphine and should not be given to patients who have become tolerant to morphine since withdrawal symptoms could result. Buprenorphine is administered sublingually in 200 mcg tablets, or by intramuscular injection (300 mcg).

Dextromoramide (Palfium)   This is a very short-acting opioid (two to three hours' duration). It is useful as an extra for occasional breakthrough pain or before a painful procedure.

Pentazocine (Fortral)   Pentazocine, a partial opioid agonist/ antagonist, is used to relieve moderate to severe pain. It is administered orally, 25–100 mg after food, or by subcutaneous, intramuscular, or intravenous injection, 30–60 mg. Rectal suppositories (50 mg) are also available. Side effects include mild respiratory depression, nausea, vomiting, dizziness, and hallucinations.

Dextropropoxyphene hydrochloride and paracetamol (Co-proxamol) This is a frequently used compound analgesic preparation.

Intravenous opioids

In Great Britain, nurses do not usually give intravenous injections. However, in some units, they may do so when there is an agreement with medical staff. Intravenous injections of opioids are given slowly, over a three to five minute period, and the effect is almost immediate. The duration of action is, however, shorter than when an opioid is given intramuscularly.

Infusion pumps

Analgesics may be administered by means of an infusion pump. There are a number of infusion pumps available for use in different situations. Routes of administration also may vary depending on the situation. Intravenous analgesic infusions may be used in the management of postoperative pain, whereas subcutaneous infusion is more usually used in palliative care. With the latter, the cannula may be placed in the chest, upper arm, or abdomen. Epidural infusions are useful in the management of acute pain, for example labour pain or postoperative pain, and preoperatively prior to amputation in an attempt to reduce postoperative phantom pain. For information on infusion sets, care of the skin, and how to use portable infusion pumps, the reader is referred to Latham (1990).

Patient-controlled analgesia Patient-controlled analgesic therapy (PACAT) is a method of intravenous opioid administration suitable for adults who are rational and not in circulatory shock. It requires purpose-built equipment in which a previously programmed drug injector is connected to a venous cannula in the patient's arm or hand. A preset dose of opioid (e.g., 2–3 mg of morphine) can then be delivered over a predetermined time, when the patient feels the need for it, by the patient himself activating a press-button switch. In one study where this method was used postoperatively, patients experienced better pain relief than would have occurred with conventional intramuscular administration, and respiratory depression was not found to be a problem (Keeri-Szanto and Heaman, 1972). In addition, it has been reported that patients are enthusiastic about the method and that side-effects are minimal (Tamsen et al., 1982). Different manufacturers provide different options with patient-controlled analgesic pumps. Some require attachment to an intravenous infusion, while others can be used while a patient is ambulatory.

Counteracting respiratory depressant effects of narcotics

Naloxone is the drug most commonly used to counteract respiratory depression. Care should be taken not to precipitate withdrawal symptoms and not to counteract all the analgesia afforded by the opioid. The suggested dose is 100–200 µg (1.5–3 µg/kg), adjusted according to the response of the patient, and then 100 µg every two minutes. The nurse must continue to observe a patient following administration of naloxone as the duration of action of this drug may be as short as 30 minutes, whereas the depressant effects of some opioids may be considerably longer. Repeated treatments with naloxone may therefore be required.

Generally speaking, it is safe to give a patient enough opioid to relieve pain but, unfortunately, many patients suffer unrelieved pain due to the inadequate use of opioid analgesics. This may be for a variety of reasons, including underprescribing, failure to understand the importance of the individual nature of pain, and, in the treatment of acute pain and the pain of terminal illness, a misplaced fear of addiction.

Non-opioid analgesics

Non-opioid analgesics such as aspirin and paracetamol are useful in the relief of musculoskeletal pain and most types of moderate to mild pain, and as an adjunct prescription for pain from bone secondaries in patients with malignant disease.

Aspirin   Aspirin has an anti-inflammatory action and acts quickly. One difficulty with this analgesic is gastric irritation, but buffered preparations that are less irritant are available. It should not be given to patients with gastrointestinal problems, to patients with haemophilia or to those who are on anticoagulant therapy, since irritation can be sufficient to cause gastric haemorrhage. The dose is 300–900 mg every four to six hours when necessary. The maximum daily dose is 4 g.

Paracetamol   This drug is similar in effect to aspirin but it has no anti-inflammatory action. It is less irritant to the gastrointestinal tract than aspirin. Overdose may cause liver damage which may not be obvious for up to six days. The dose is 0.5–1 g, either in the form of tablets or as an elixir.

Diflunisal (Dolobid)   The contraindications for this drug are the same as for aspirin. The dose is 250–500 mg. Tablets should be swallowed whole. Absorption is reduced if the drug is given in conjunction with an antacid.

Mefenamic acid (Ponstan)   This drug is used to treat mild to moderate pain. It should not be given to patients with peptic ulceration or inflammatory conditions of the bowel, to those with renal or hepatic impairment or to pregnant women. It may cause drowsiness, dizziness, gastric disturbances, and diarrhoea. The dose is 500 mg taken orally after food.

Ibuprofen   Ibuprofen is used in the treatment of pain and inflammation in rheumatic disease and other musculoskeletal disorders. The dose is 200–400 mg given orally in tablet form.

Diclofenac sodium (Voltarol)   is used to treat renal colic and biliary colic. It can be given IM or by suppository, and should not cause drowsiness.

Carbamazepine (Tegretol) Although not strictly an analgesic, this drug is very effective in the treatment of trigeminal neuralgia.

Amytryptyline is a tricyclic antidepressant drug and works as an adjuvant in certain nerve pains.

Other drugs

New preparations are constantly appearing on the market, and it is important that nurses appreciate the action of new drugs and know about possible side-effects. Detailed information can be found in pharmacology textbooks. The British National Formulary gives up-to-date information, and nurses should be familiar with consulting this.

The management of acute pain using analgesic drugs

In treating acute pain a preventive approach is useful. Analgesics may be given before pain returns to prevent severe pain. Analgesics should, however, be viewed as part of an overall pain-control strategy that includes a variety of measures, some of which may be taught to the patient. In individualizing management of acute pain, the nurse should observe a patient's response to a treatment and be prepared to discuss possible adjustments in dose if analgesics are being given.

Intramuscular or intravenous routes may be used for severe pain, changing to oral, sublingual, or rectal routes when the intensity of the pain subsides. The choice of route depends on the medication prescribed and on the nature of the injury or operation site. However, nurses should recognize the dangers of changing to less potent analgesics too soon. When an analgesic is not effective in terms of duration of pain, then shortening the interval between administrations may be of help rather than adding a drug to sedate.

Sometimes it is helpful to give an opioid along with a non-opioid analgesic. When opioids are in use, an opioid antagonist such as naloxone should always be available should opioid-induced respiratory depression develop. Nurses should always be aware of the possibility of undertreating pain and the importance of frequent assessment with the patient.

The fear of addiction is not well founded in the treatment of acute pain with opioids. Undertreatment may in fact increase the likelihood of 'clock-watching' – when a patient waits expectantly for the next dose of analgesia. This kind of situation can lead to psychological problems. The answer to avoiding this lies in providing adequate pain control.

Accident and emergency treatment   For relief of acute pain, particularly in a casualty department, Entonox (a 50/50 mixture of nitrous oxide and oxygen from one cylinder) may be used advantageously. It is rapidly effective and can be self-administered.

The management of chronic pain using analgesics and other drugs

The management of chronic pain presents an entirely different problem. Patients suffering chronic pain fall into two groups. First, those suffering persistent pain with a normal expectation of life and, second, those who have a short expectation of life and are suffering from malignant disease. In the latter case, pain is continuous and becomes worse. Because of the short life expectancy, the possibility of addiction to opioids is not important. These patients should be given analgesia in sufficient strength, quantity, and frequency to control their pain (Lipton, 1979; Twycross and Lack, 1983).

It is increasingly common practice in palliative medicine to use the guidelines of the WHO for the relief of cancer pain. If after assessment of the patient drug therapy is decided upon, four categories of basic drugs are used. These are non-opioids such as aspirin or paracetamol, or non-steroidal anti-inflammatory drugs such as Ibuprofen; second, weak opioids such as codeine or dextropoxyphene, third, strong opioids such as morphine, pethidine, or buprenorphine. The fourth category is adjuvants, which include drugs like anticonvulsants such as carbamazipine, and neuroleptics such as prochlorperazine and haloperidol; anxiolytics such as diazepam; antidepressants such as amitriptyline, and corticosteroids such as prednisolone.

These drugs are administered 'by the clock' and 'by the ladder'. In other words, one starts with the non-opioid drugs and adds adjuvant drugs if indicated. One then ascends the ladder to the weak opioids, which may be given either alone or in combination with non-opioids and adjuvants. If pain persists, strong opioids with or without non-opioids or adjuvants are given. It is important that at each stage the patient and his pain are reassessed. Further information can be found in Cancer Pain Relief (WHO). The nurse should also consult the British National Formulary, updated each year for information on side-effects associated with the above-mentioned drugs.

In the case of non-malignant pain, it is wise to use drugs that do not have abuse potential, combined with other relief measures aimed at increasing the quality of the patient's life. Sometimes, psychotropic drugs, especially antidepressants and phenothiazines, may relieve chronic pain. Amitriptyline, for example, may reduce the severity and frequency of migraine.

Transcutaneous electric nerve stimulation (TENS)

TENS can be used for the relief of both acute and chronic pain. The mechanism by which TENS results in pain relief is not understood, although there have been a number of suggested explanations. Some people feel that TENS acts by activating nerve endings in the same way as the application of heat or cold. One possibility is that stimulating large-diameter nerve fibres closes the gate (Chapter 2) to the transmission of pain impulses (Nathan and Wall, 1974). Other suggestions are that TENS acts by blocking primary afferent nerve fibres, or by stimulating the production of endorphins, the body's own naturally occurring opiate-like substances.

There are many kinds of electrical devices for TENS. These include small models, designed for patients to use themselves, which have a clip so they can be attached to a belt or put in a pocket.

A TENS system basically consists of a battery-powered electronic pulse generator to which are connected two to four lead wires ending in electrodes that are placed on the skin.

Nurses should be acquainted with the use of TENS because they are ideally placed both in hospital and community settings to help and advise patients regarding its use. Patients with chronic pain often find a TENS machine helpful, sometimes in conjunction with other therapies. The machine should be positioned so that the patient finds it easy to adjust the controls.

The positioning of the electrodes is important. They are usually placed over the area of a peripheral nerve innervating the painful site. The best place may be nearest to the pain, but sometimes the patient may find relief when the electrodes are placed away from the painful site. Different patients report different effects from the use of TENS. Some patients only find relief from pain during stimulation while others may report periods of relief following treatment. These differences may reflect the differences in the nature of their pain. Patients need therefore to adjust the controls according to their own needs. The stimulation is felt by the patient as a tingling or buzzing sensation and this can be adjusted by the knobs on the side of the unit. The patient can adjust the sensation until it is pleasant and relieves the pain. Some electrodes need an application of conductive gel. Self-adhesive electrodes are now available and are becoming more popular. There are reusable ones as well as disposable ones. A patient can wear the unit for as little time or as long as he likes. The electrodes can be left in place and the leads reattached when necessary. Sometimes the skin may become irritated and changing the tape used to keep the electrodes in place may help. If a rash occurs from the gel, then another type of gel should be substituted.

TENS may be used to treat all types of chronic pain, but the results are variable. Some patients experience complete relief while others have none. TENS may also be used for relief of postoperative pain. Sterile, pre-gelled electrodes may be placed close to a wound and left in place. A stimulator can then be connected when required. Deep breathing, coughing, and moving may be facilitated by the use of a TENS unit and may reduce the need for opioid analgesia. If a TENS unit is to be used postoperatively it is useful if the patient can be made familiar with it prior to surgery. TENS is also useful in labour pain.

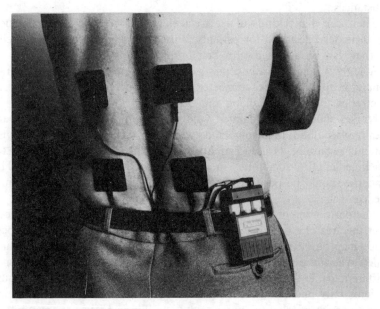

Application of TENS. (Photograph courtesy of Spembly Medical.)

Acupuncture analgesia

Acupuncture is a system of medicine developed by the ancient Chinese. During acupuncture treatment, fine needles pierce the skin at certain points on the body where particular effects can be obtained. The needles may be rotated or stimulated.

The Chinese explanation of how acupuncture analgesia works is based on the idea that life force flows around certain lines on the body known as meridians. Needling points on these lines is thought to correct an abnormal flow of life forces (Mann, 1971). Another explanation that has been suggested is that acupuncture stimulates the production of endorphins (Mayer *et al.*, 1976).

Some acupuncturists use traditional Chinese acupuncture points which may not necessarily be near the site of pain. Other acupuncturists use trigger points, which are small very sensitive regions in the muscle or connective tissue. They may be in the area of the pain or at some distance from it. Sometimes trigger points and acupuncture points correspond.

Pressure and massage on trigger points may relieve pain. Some therapists try using acupuncture points in this way, rather than needling the points. This is called acupressure. Illustrations of acupuncture points are shown in other publications (Mann, 1971; McCaffery, 1983).

Acupuncture analgesia may be helpful in relieving chronic pain and has been found to be particularly useful in the treatment of migraine (Lipton, 1979). It is not effective in treating advanced cancer pain.

Nerve blocks

In certain circumstances, perhaps when other methods of pain relief are contraindicated or have proved ineffective, and where pain is unilateral and restricted to a particular area, a local nerve block may be considered. In this procedure, the conduction of the nerve impulses which give rise to pain is prevented by injecting a local anaesthetic which produces a temporary effect, or a drug that destroys the nerve fibres (neurolytic agent), such as phenol, producing a longer-term effect.

Nerve blocks are carried out by doctors, usually anaesthetists, but the nurse should play a supportive role before and during the procedure, and should also be aware of possible complications, some of which are specific to different types of nerve block. For example, following epidural anaesthesia there may be urinary retention. After any phenol injection, the exact position of the patient, as specified by the doctor, is crucial and should be maintained for one hour. In addition, observation of the patient for signs of hypotension and haematoma is obligatory for two hours after the procedure. Local anaesthetic blocks may be effective for up to 12–18 hours, whereas a phenol block may be effective for 8–22 weeks. The use of nerve blocks for the relief of chronic pain is discussed by Latham (1983).

Summary

- It is best to treat pain using combined physical and psychological treatments.
- There are several therapies lying within the province of the nurse, such as distraction, guided imagery, and relaxation.
- There may be some degree of overlap between therapies.
- The quality of the nurse–patient relationship will influence the patient's willingness to try a particular technique.
- Sometimes health professionals doubt a patient's pain if the patient is able to distract himself.
- Distraction may be a potent pain reliever.
- Imagery may be used in conjunction with relaxation.
- Visual imagery can be helpful during uncomfortable procedures.
- Several techniques are available to achieve a state of relaxation, for example meditation, yoga or progressive relaxation exercises.
- A quiet environment and comfortable position are recommended for practising relaxation.
- Instructions for practising relaxation may be recorded by the nurse on a tape for a patient.
- Analgesic drugs are commonly used for relief of pain.
- Opioid analgesics are usually the only effective drugs in combating severe pain.
- The most commonly used opioid analgesic is morphine.
- Naloxone is the drug most commonly used to counteract opioid-induced respiratory depression.
- Patient-controlled analgesia is one method suitable for adults who are rational and not in circulatory shock.
- A preventive approach is useful in treating acute pain.
- Patients with a short life expectancy should be given sufficient analgesia in terms of strength, quantity, and frequency to control their pain.
- Patients who suffer pain of non-malignant origin may be treated with drugs that do not have abuse potential, combined with other pain therapies.
- TENS may be used for relief of either acute or chronic pain but the results are variable in accordance with the type of pain and its location.
- Acupuncture analgesia may be used in the area of pain or at trigger or traditional acupuncture points.
- In certain circumstances, doctors may carry out nerve blocks to relieve patients' pain, and nurses should be aware of their supportive role to

patients and any possible complications that may occur with this type of treatment.

References

British National Formulary, No. 20 (1990) British Medical Association and The Pharmaceutical Society of Great Britain.

Copp, L. (1974) The spectrum of suffering, *American Journal of Nursing*, 74(3):491–5.

Jaffe, J. H. (1975) Drug addiction and drug abuse, in *The Pharmacological Basis of Therapeutics* (eds L. S. Goodman and M. Gilman) (5th edn), Macmillan, pp. 284–324.

Johnson, D. and Spielberger, C. (1968) The effects of relaxation training and the passage of time on measures of state and trait anxiety, *Journal of Clinical Psychology*, 24:20.

Keeri-Szanto, M. and Heaman, S. (1972) Postoperative demand analgesia, *Surgery, Gynecology and Obstetrics*, 134:647–51.

Latham, J. (1983) 1. The pain relief team, *Nursing Times* (27 April):54–7; 2. The nervous system, *Nursing Times* (4 May):57–60; 3. Complications, *Nursing Times* (11 May):36–8; 4. The nurse's role, *Nursing Times* (18 May):33–5.

Latham, J. (1990) *Pain Control*. Austen Cornish Ltd with The Lisa Sainsbury Foundation.

Lipton, S. (1979) Treatment of chronic pain, Chapter 10, *The Control of Chronic Pain*, Edward Arnold.

Mann, F. (ed.) (1971) *Acupuncture: The Ancient Chinese Art of Healing*, Heinemann.

Mayer, D. J., Price, D. D. and Raffii, A. (1976) Antagonism of acupuncture analgesia in man by the narcotic antagonist naloxone, *Brain Research*, 121:368–77.

McCaffery, M. (1983) *Nursing the Patient in Pain*, Harper & Row.

Melzack, R. and Wall, P. D. (1982) *The Challenge of Pain*, Penguin Books.

Nathan, P. W. and Wall, P. D. (1974) Treatment of postherpetic neuralgia by prolonged electric stimulation, *British Medical Journal*, 3:645–7.

Tamsen, A., Hartvig, P., Fagerlund, C., Dahlström, B. and Bondesson, U. (1982) Patient controlled analgesic therapy: Clinical experience, *Acta Anaesthesiologica Scandinavica*, Supplement 74:157–60.

Twycross, R. G. and Lack, S. A. (1983) *Symptom Control in Far Advanced Cancer Pain Relief*, Pitman.

Wiener, C. L. (1975) Pain assessment on an orthopaedic ward. *Nursing Outlook*, 23:508–16.

8

Feelings about pain

I am resentful against the hospital because they [the staff] should have
warned you about how to cope and about what was going to happen and
what you were going to go through.

(Patient after discharge from hospital)

Feelings of patients

Negative feelings related to unrelieved acute pain may impede a patient's
recovery and delay rehabilitation. In addition, patients may view the
prospect of any future hospitalization with anxiety and trepidation. For
example, one patient said that if she had to go into hospital again, 'I
would be awfully anxious, extremely anxious and, I mean, I really
couldn't go through taking that pain again. It was terrible. I just
wouldn't go in again if I knew something similar was to happen to me.'
Later, when asked if despite her extreme anxiety she felt that she would
have a little more courage to ask for information for herself, she replied,
'Yes, I think I would. I don't think I would sort of freeze up when
everybody comes round the bed and looks at you. I think I would be able
to ask exactly what was happening and what they were doing rather than
just leave it and not have them tell me a thing.'

Patients suffering chronic pain are in a different position, but they
may also be affected by initial inadequate treatment, although the
situation may be more tolerable if at least those around these patients are
interested in them as people. So often patients suffering chronic pain are
referred back and forth from specialist to specialist. A number may be
referred to a pain relief clinic, where they will find an interested doctor
and/or nurse and, depending on the local organization, perhaps a
multidisciplinary team.

Most patients who have suffered pain appreciate an outlet for
expression of the feelings, whether they are being cared for at home, in a
hospital ward, or as an outpatient. The needs of patients vary according

to the characteristics of their pain. Patients who have experienced unrelieved acute pain may feel that ventilation of feelings on one or a few occasions may spur them along the road to recovery. Patients experiencing unrelieved chronic benign pain may require frequent sessions to help them to come to terms with living with pain and to guide them towards an increased quality of life. For patients who have the pain of malignant disease there is the deepest suffering – what Cecily Saunders (1967) has called 'total pain' – a combination of physical, emotional, social, and spiritual suffering.

The feelings patients experience when pain is not relieved vary with personality, previous pain experiences, expectations of the health carers and available therapies. It is important for health carers to realize that patients often need help to express these feelings, and that patients may experience great relief simply on being made to feel free to do this. However, nurses should not force the issue but facilitate natural expressions of feelings.

Aftermath of pain

When pain is relieved, or brought under control, patients sometimes still appreciate the opportunity to express feelings about the effects of pain when it was not controlled. When the cause of pain is removed, the patient needs to be told this. For example, following a painful procedure such as a sternomarrow puncture, patients might find it easier to relax once they know this. On the other hand, the nurse should not tell the patient that a procedure is over and that there is no possibility of further discomfort until she is sure that this is so, since a second attempt at the procedure may be required.

Some patients need to know that their behaviour while in pain was acceptable and normal. A feeling of having lost control may lessen a person's self-esteem. One patient said, 'I felt I had to apologize to the nursing staff for my behaviour but I was in such agony.' (In this particular case the analgesia provided had been inadequate.) Sometimes it helps patients to know that other people react in a similar way. Efforts to raise self-esteem following painful experiences may be very worthwhile in preventing lingering anxiety and emotional feelings.

When pain is only partially controlled, some patients may be relieved and express this, whereas others may experience feelings of fatigue from accumulated pain. Some prefer to forget about the pain and try to put it at the back of their minds. Others do not forget so easily, and encouragement to express pent up feelings may help.

When patients who have suffered chronic pain recognize that

improvement has occurred, they may have problems adjusting to former activities. In helping such a patient, it is useful to remember that social, physical and financial changes may have occurred during the time he suffered. Added to this are personality changes brought about by despair and depression. Prolonged pain may leave a person feeling isolated and angry with the world. Rehabilitation may require assistance and understanding from the nurse so that the patient can regain former confidence and increase his joy of living. Life may never be as it was formerly; efforts to help the patient to express his feelings about this may help him progress to new ways of fulfilment.

Feelings of nursing staff

Nursing provides the opportunity to develop natural nurturing skills, but for many the job is a stressful one. Many nurses develop feelings of powerlessness and frustration when they are unable to relieve suffering and may blame themselves or others. Unfortunately, when a nurse does become stressed (for this reason or any of a number of other reasons that make the job a stressful one), there may be a tendency for colleagues to assume that she cannot cope.

It has been pointed out (Latimer, 1980) that it is difficult being involved so closely on a day-to-day basis with other people's suffering. One student nurse wrote about the experience of working on a ward where all the staff had been involved in the programme about pain management mentioned in the preface of this book. She said, 'It was rewarding to be involved in a team where there was open discussion about individual patients' pain relief'. She later contrasted this to a ward where she was subsequently working and felt frustrated at the lack of awareness among members of staff.

A student who had attended several lectures on the nursing management of pain subsequently went to work in a casualty department and was distressed by the following incident:

A man arrived with chest pain, a possible myocardial infarction. On his arrival the care area was very busy; his initial recordings were carried out but he had to wait about 1½ hours before any decision was made as to what ward he should go to. Meanwhile, his relatives were waiting round the corner in a waiting area, obviously very worried about his condition. The patient was ashen white, sweating and obviously in a considerable amount of distress.

Another student nurse was very unhappy about a certain event when on night duty. A third-year nurse was on night duty with her at the time. The student nurse commented:

A patient returned from theatre and was suffering great physical and psychological pain. He was given an injection of diamorphine but this obviously was not adequate or appropriate for this man's pain. The third-year nurse informed the night sister when she came around. Sister told us to wait half-an-hour and if the patient's condition had not improved to inform the doctor. Meanwhile the patient's pain was not relieved.

Birch (1979) has also noted that failure to relieve pain is one cause of stress in student nurses. In order not to face the discomfort that a patient's suffering evokes in a nurse, the sense of powerlessness may result in nurses avoiding the patient. This is an attempt to shut off the reality of the failure and guilt on the part of the nurse. Accumulation of these feelings of frustration and powerlessness may lead to depression and, in some cases, great unhappiness. Nurses may even leave nursing due to lack of job satisfaction.

For the patient, prolonged pain is demoralizing and frightening. If carers avoid him he may become withdrawn and preoccupied with his pain. It is important that the nurse spends time with the patient and acknowledges the reality of his pain. Indicating that she is willing to stay with him and face the pain with him will be of great support and comfort. This is one constructive way of handling the feelings aroused in a nurse when she cares for a patient whose pain she cannot alleviate.

In the care of the terminally ill patient, a nurse may fear being the one who administers the last dose of analgesic before death. This can be particularly distressing if it has been necessary to increase the dose of opioid to control the pain, since the nurse may feel that she is in some way responsible for the patient's death. This distress is understandable, and colleagues should be supportive of each other in such situations.

Nurses' stress may also be relieved by more open discussion of feelings in the ward situation. Nurse teachers should encourage learners to approach trained staff in a constructive way about issues that are concerning them, and trained staff should be encouraged to acquire the skills necessary to deal sensitively with such situations. Another aspect of the problem is the task of raising awareness in all levels of staff regarding the importance of pain management in general. This is an area for discussion within continuing education and must be given priority.

One way of learning about feelings

Sometimes it may be difficult for nurses to understand the feelings of patients who experience pain and to understand their own feelings in relation to providing pain relief.

The following exercise in role play is one that we tried out in the research project that led to writing this book. The participants were nurses who worked in surgical wards, but it has been used in classroom situations as well. Nurses could initiate this role play themselves. Alternatively, a ward sister or clinical teacher might like to use the idea.

Role play is a valuable aid to learning and one way in which learners may be encouraged to explore their attitudes to pain. However, its use should always be supervised, in the first instance at least, by experienced teachers. Care should also be taken for participants to adopt pseudo-names and always for them to be deroled at the conclusion. A minimum of six people in the group is recommended, with no limitations on the maximum number, as those not actually role playing act as observers. The exercise is in two parts with two separate themes. The players are each briefed in private.

Part 1. A participant is asked to act out the role of a patient in severe pain. The other player is given the role of a disbelieving, busy nurse. The players are allowed to act the situation, until it spontaneously concludes (average time five minutes). Following the conclusion of the role play, each player is asked to relate her feelings in the role. These are noted on a blackboard if one is available. Finally, each player is deroled by each one saying who she is in real life and not the role she played. Observers are requested not to discuss their observations among themselves. Part 2 of the exercise is then commenced.

Part 2. Two participants are again required and each is briefed privately. One person is asked to act the role of a patient in severe pain and the other of a nurse who believes the patient. The role play continues until it concludes spontaneously (average time two minutes). Each role player is asked how she feels and the comments are recorded as before. Participants are then deroled.

Following the role play, observers are asked for their comments on the nature of these interactions and a comparison is made.

Try out the above exercise and then compare your findings with ours (Figure 8.1). (I have found it best to choose a particularly sympathetic nurse for the role of the disbeliever in Part 1. In this way the group can be supportive of her later, knowing that she would never behave like that in real life.)

This exercise may sound simple, but it has been valuable in its simplicity because it demonstrates very clearly to nurses the implications of patient–nurse interactions. It is thought-provoking to consider the effects that nurses themselves can create in a learning situation using role play.

Some points usually noted by observers	Theme 1	Theme 2
Length of time of interactions	Long	Short
Tone of voices used	High pitched and fast	Calm
Non-verbal clues	No touching	Touching
	No eye-to-eye contact	Eye-to-eye contact
	Nurse stands	Same level
Feelings of nurse	Anger	Sympathy
	Insecurity	Responsibility
	Powerlessness	Autonomy
Feelings of patient	Anger	Empathy
	Frustration	Concern on his behalf
	Powerlessness	Involvement

Figure 8.1 Role play

Several nurses have said of this exercise, 'It makes you think.' As Bond (1979) has stated:

> Where nurses have been taught to understand patients' pain and to deal with it by physical and psychological means, patients express a much greater degree of satisfaction with treatment than where the staff have not received any training of this kind.

Summary

- Negative feelings related to unrelieved acute pain may impede a patient's recovery.
- Most patients appreciate being allowed to express their feelings.
- Patients may need encouragement to express feelings.
- When improvement has occurred, patients may need help to adjust to former activities.
- Nurses sometimes develop feelings of powerlessness and frustration when they are unable to relieve suffering.
- Nurses' stress may be relieved when open discussion is encouraged.
- Role play may help nurses in understanding their own feelings and those of patients.
- *Patients are more satisfied when nurses have been taught about understanding pain.*

References

Birch, J. (1979) The anxious learners, *Nursing Mirror*, **148**, 17–22.

Bond, M. J. (Editor) (1979) The influence of learning and the environment on pain, in *Pain, Its Nature, Analysis and Treatment*, Churchill Livingstone.

Latimer, J. (1980) Stress and the student nurse, *Nursing*, **10**, 449–50.

Saunders, C. (1967) *The Management of Terminal Illness*, Hospital Medical Publications.

9

The role of nursing in pain management – some thoughts for the future

> But pain is a perfect miserie, the worst of all evils an excessive overturns all patience.
>
> *(Paradise Lost,* Milton)
>
> But pain is a perfect misery, the worst of all evils, an excessive overturns all *patients.*
>
> (Sofaer, 1992)

Much progress has been made in recent years in techniques to relieve pain. Many words have been spoken, and many articles and books have been published. Still, people suffer pain. Even when many techniques have been tried, patients often return to pain clinics and report they still have pain. Even after wise people have spoken at conferences and published in reputable journals, people still suffer pain.

What may be difficult to understand is why so many scientists, therapists, physicians, and others who acknowledge pain and its expression as a subjective phenomenon, sometimes tend to forget that each individual who experiences pain also has a unique set of *life* experiences that go hand-in-hand with the pain. These events and experiences, past and present, need to be explored in the *context* of the pain, alongside therapeutic interventions, if and when appropriate.

Pain cannot be set apart from other events in life. Acute pain may have a foreseeable end, but its interpretation and meaning for a patient is in the context of his own framework, and not of *ours.* The person who suffers chronic pain will see his pain in the context of his life events; past, present and possibly future; the person who is at the end of life and in pain will be searching for peace of mind, along with pain relief.

Most nurses intuitively realize these facts and are well placed, in fact, I would venture, best placed, to help assess and to assist all pain sufferers. What is needed in the nursing profession is the confidence and skills to implement support for patients, knowledge regarding the wide range of techniques and therapies that exist, and the ability to communicate effectively with medical colleagues for the benefit of patients. Arthur Kleinman (1988), in his moving book *The Illness Narratives*, comments that in relation to case conferences where multidisciplinary teams were discussing the pain of patients, 'the nurses, physiotherapists, occupational therapists and social worker often had more important information to contribute than did the medical specialist, but they clearly occupied a lower status and were overruled by the pain experts.'

This introductory book is intended to encourage nurses and other health professionals to further their thoughts and ideas on how best to help people who suffer pain. It is worth pointing out that no textbook can provide us with the experience to cope either with pain itself or with the pain of others, and that so-called 'physical pain' is not an entity removed from psychological anguish, although people express it and cope with it in diverse ways.

Pain *is* a complex phenomenon experienced in the context of the complexity of human nature. Chronic pain particularly throws that normal complexity further into chaos and may produce crisis situations for the sufferer. Pain clinics, developed to try and sort out 'the problems' operate in different ways, some being staffed by a variety of specialists ranging from consultant anaesthetists and a team of psychologists and other specialists providing a range of therapies, to other clinics operating at a more humble level.

What is important, no matter where pain is being treated, is the attitude and understanding towards patients. Finer (1991) utilizes the concept of 'a pain culture' – the values of patients and health professionals expressed towards each other by virtue of the worlds they live in. The patient lives in a world of pain, and the language he uses to express his living is derived from that world. The doctors and nurses, on the other hand, are well and not 'in pain'. (Although they may well suffer the 'anguish' of failure to help others.) Somehow, or other, for empathy and understanding to develop, both patient and health carer have to understand the world of the other. Pain therapy therefore has to be based on shared responsibility between patient and therapist. What complicates the issue further is that often several therapies may be tried out, and so communication and understanding has to develop between the health carers themselves. This takes time, requires an understanding of each other's qualities, attributes and skills, and, in order to be of benefit to patients, has to be well co-ordinated. This applies both in acute and chronic settings.

Nurses unfortunately still have a way to go before defining a role for themselves in all of this. On the other hand, many nurses though are experienced 'therapists' without realizing it, and others may need additional help with education to boost confidence in developing skills. What is beginning to happen, though, in nursing is the realization, with theoretical backing (to some people it has always been commonsense), that a human being goes through different stages of life and development, is subject to ups and downs, and has a role in controlling his own life. This realization is *crucial* to the management of pain, for it is the control of the balance between pain and pleasant feelings that makes life liveable and bearable for some, and the lack of control that makes life and living intolerable and unbearable for others. For those who have lost control, helping them to restore the balance may involve the acceptance by people who suffer chronic pain that pain and pleasant feelings may coexist. In other words, 'living with the pain' – a phrase much used and abused, misunderstood, and brandished about. It should be interpreted as meaning living a life that involves positive feelings about oneself and the world, as well as having the pain. This is difficult for many people to accept; they want the pain doctor and the nurse to 'take it away'.

The following are a couple of excerpts of work with patients in pain clinics, and illustrate the kinds of things patients say they feel.

Mrs Q is a 57-year-old lady who has suffered back pain for many years. She says that she feels 'isolated'. Her husband has recently taken early retirement to 'look after her'. Her typical day begins at 7.30 am when she has a cup of tea brought to her in bed. She then gets up, and after getting dressed lies down again because she 'feels too weak with the exhaustion of having got dressed'. After a while she potters about the house. After lunch she lies down again. She has been married for 38 years, but it is a 'long time since lovemaking has taken place'. She has not been to a shop 'for several years'. She does her shopping by catalogue. She had a friend who used to visit her, but no longer feels she has any friends. She says it is several years since she has gone out except to the hospital, which takes several days of preparation. 'I admit', she says, 'that the pain has taken over my life; it is bigger in my mind than it need be'. Mrs Q was encouraged to go for little walks starting with three minutes and building up to one hour over a period of a month. She was encouraged to think about the areas of her life she would like to improve, and especially to give thought to her personal and social situation. She agreed to setting some short-term goals to increase her quality of life. She started by taking short walks, but because she found she really could do it, she had a tendency to overdo the activity and required further advice and counselling.

Mr N is in his late 70s. He has experienced the Second World War. He lives with his wife and they have a harmonious and warm relationship. They cry together sometimes with frustration about the pain. He experiences back pain and is unable to walk for long periods, or to sit at the table and eat in comfort, and feels quite unable to participate in any social life. When asked what he would like to talk about, Mr N looked back over his life; when asked what he felt was shaping and colouring his life situation at the present time, he talked in great detail about the death and funeral of a relative many years ago. After some 40 minutes of reminiscing, he finally said, 'I know I am digging my own grave'. In consultation with his wife, it was decided that Mr N would begin to take note of the positive things in his life, and with her help they would recall the good times together. Mr and Mrs N, with the encouragement of the author, drew up a set of distractions to help Mr N focus on more positive aspects of his life.

A final note on the experience of chronic pain

This book has addressed the issues of relationship between psychological factors and pain, cultural dimensions of pain expression, accountability and responsibility of nurses, communication between health professionals and patients, an introduction to pain therapies, and a few vignettes from the lives of patients the author has met.

So what is left? The reader may well ask. Well, quite a lot really. For a start, this book has not addressed the complex aspects associated with the physiology of pain (the reader is referred to suitable material), and second, and probably more important for the nurse, is the issue of *what* to do in the 'here-and-now' when faced with a patient in pain when attempted control of the pain has failed. This is particularly important for a patient suffering chronic pain, for this is where we often come unstuck and feel a sense of failure.

It may be useful to take your clue from the patient. Start where the patient starts. In the experience of the author, patients sometimes start to talk at the point where they want to express 'isolation' and 'fear'. If a patient can be allowed to express this he may show strong emotions associated with present or past experiences, and associated with a feeling of a lack of ability to build a bridge for himself to enhance the quality of life and living. If one is to help build that bridge, the nurse should guard against preconceived ideas, as so often medical colleagues and others refer to patients with pain as having 'emotional overlay'. This is due to a *lack* of acceptance by some professionals that emotionality is *naturally* associated with the pain experience, an idea that people outside the world of nursing and medicine seem to have no difficulty with.

A major problem, however, is when inexperienced carers find themselves dealing with complicated and difficult emotional problems. Of course, there is a wide variation in how people express feelings, and not everyone wants to or feels it appropriate to 'let it all hang out' with a stranger. This must be respected. However, generally speaking, people who suffer chronic pain often appreciate a sympathetic ear, which may be the first step for the patient in trying to recreate a positive image of himself and his world. If we are to be of real benefit to our patients who suffer pain, then it is essential to develop ways of assessing individual emotional responses, and to assist patients subsequently in developing coping strategies.

Do not underestimate your own first step either. We all learn by experience – but perhaps it might be helpful to have a few hints of what to expect. Sometimes patients like to talk about the past and what they used to be able to do. (One young woman patient with multiple injuries following a road traffic accident talked much about her past, particularly her sports activities, and it took several sessions before she would concentrate on the present or even give a thought to the future). The kinds of feelings expressed often include sadness, despair, anger, grief, and the numbness of silence. Lonesomeness and isolation, especially if a person lives alone, may compound the situation. But these may be present too in a person who does not live alone, but feels isolated because of pain. One patient expressed this feeling as being the most difficult to cope with because she felt trapped in a marriage of 38 years with a husband who 'humiliated' her because he did not believe her pain.

The nurse, then, is often faced with the situation of how to 'enter the world' of another person's pain. The one thing that can be said that applies to *all* situations is that you should try to make *good contact* with the patient.

'What does it feel like? Pain and more pain.
Darkness and silence and pain. Constant pain.
And no one can reach me . . . no one has the sympathy,
the wisdom, the courage, to find their way inside.

My wilderness of pain.

To find the right words.
Or maybe you, for *you've* helped me speak
('David', Jerusalem, 1984)

It is the nurse who must have courage, and to exercise it to the best advantage it is wise to find out as much as possible through reading, attending seminars, and sharing problems with colleagues.

Sometimes nurses ask how it is possible to enter the world of another's pain and remain uninvolved emotionally. A non-nursing colleague approached the author during the writing of this book and asked if nurses are taught to 'remain professional'. 'If only they would come closer to her' (referring to his elderly infirm mother), 'if only they would touch her, if only they would hold her hand.' He was reassured that in fact nurses are encouraged to touch, and to hold a hand.

People express their feelings in different ways and it must be said that one should not push another into emotional expression but be guided by the sufferer. Many nurses perhaps find it easier to hold someone who is distraught and to cry with a person in consolation than to deal with angry feelings. It is important to remember that there is no right way to say anything, and that if you are stuck and do not know what to say, then be honest and say so.

Remember too the power of non-verbal communication and the words of Socrates: '*Nobility and dignity, self-abasement and servility, prudence and understanding, insolence and vulgarity, are all reflected in the face and in the attitudes of the body whether still or in motion.*' This equally applies to nurses as well as to patients.

I think it is fitting towards the end of this chapter and of this book to quote the late Professor John Heimler, a man who spent most of his life helping others to cross the bridge from an unhappy and painful past to a positive present and hope for the future:

Do not ask 'why' pain, only what has to be done with it.

(*The Storm*, John Heimler)

On a more lighthearted note . . .

Some years ago the author was due to give a series of lectures at a London teaching hospital, and arrived at King's Cross Station three hours late. It was a very hot day. Feeling rather harassed, she took a taxi and found herself in the company of a very chatty taxi driver. In the middle of a traffic-jam he quizzed her about her profession and her reason for going to the hospital. On revealing that she was about to lecture on pain, the taxi driver turned off the engine, threw his hands in the air, and shouted at the top of his voice, 'I know *all* about pain, when the pain's gorne, it doesn't 'urt anymore!'

Let humanity ever be our goal.

Goethe

Good luck!

References

Finer, B. (1991) Personal communication.
Kleinman, A. (1988) *The Illness Narratives*. Basic Books, New York.

Glossary

Acute pain An episode of pain of sudden onset, short duration and foreseeable end

Adaptation The process by which a patient may gradually manage to endure pain and carry on despite it, perhaps without obvious outward signs of pain

Analogue scale (for determining pain scores) A scale on which the extremes of pain experience (no pain, pain as bad as it can be) are indicated. The patient places a mark on the scale to represent the level of pain at the time, and the distance of this mark in standard units from the 'no pain' end of the scale is taken as the pain score

Body chart Simple outlines of the front and back views of the body on which the site of a patient's pain can be recorded

Chronic pain Pain lasting for six months or more

Deep pain Pain originating in the organs of the body. It is usually not as well localized as superficial pain and has an aching quality

Drug dependence
(a) *Psychological dependence* 'The intense craving and compulsive perpetuation of abuse to repeat the desired effect of a psychotropic drug' (World Health Organization 1969)
(b) *Physical dependence* 'An adaptive state which manifests itself by intense physical disturbances when administration of the drug is suspended or when its action is affected by the administration of a specific antagonist' (World Health Organization 1969). With continued use of morphine or heroin, physical dependence usually takes place within weeks of the first dose.

Drug tolerance The need, with long-term drug therapy, to administer increasingly large doses to produce the same effect

Opioids Drugs derived from opium. These can be synthetic or naturally derived

Pain-assessment chart A written record, usually over a period of hours or days, of the intensity and site of a patient's pain and the actions taken to control the pair

Pain autobiography   An individual's collective previous experience of pain

Pain-description chart   A list of adjectives that could be used to describe the intensity and quality of pain, used as an aid in pain assessment

Pain profile   A record (usually graphic) of a patient's pain scores, usually over a period of hours or days, used to assess the response to pain-relieving measures

Pain threshold   The least stimulus intensity at which a person perceives pain

Pain tolerance   The greatest stimulus intensity causing pain that a person is prepared to tolerate

Psychogenic pain   Pain with no detectable physical cause in a patient with a history of expressing emotional problems in terms of pain

Referred pain   Pain felt at a site other than that which has been stimulated

State anxiety   Anxiety that may be present in a patient facing a potentially stressful event

Superficial pain   Pain originating from the stimulation of the skin or mucous membranes. It may be described as bright, pricking, or burning, and is usually localized

General bibliography

Bond, M. R. (1979) *Pain: Its Nature, Analysis and Treatment*, Churchill Livingstone, Edinburgh.

Bonica, J. J. (1981) *Pain research and therapy: Past achievements and future challenges*, Presidential Address to the International Association for the Study of Pain, Edinburgh.

Boore, J. (1977) Preoperative care of patients. *Nursing Times* 73: 12, 409–11.

Boore, J. R. P. (1979) Nursing surgical patients in acute pain, *Nursing*, 1, 37–43.

Botting, J. H. (1979) Understanding analgesic drugs, *Nursing*, 2, 70–6.

British National Formulary (1990) British Medical Association and The Royal Pharmaceutical Society of Great Britain.

Cartwright, P. D. (1985) Pain control after surgery: a survey of current practice. *Annals of the Royal College of Surgeons of England* 67, 13–16.

Cancer Pain Relief (1986) World Health Organization, Geneva.

Connechen, J., Shanley, E. and Robson, H. (1982) *Pharmacology for Nurses*, Baillière Tindall.

Craig, K. D. (1975) Social modeling determinants of pain processes, *Pain*, 1, 375–8.

Davis, P. S. (1988) Changing nursing practice for more effective control of post operative pain through a staff initiated educational programme. *Nurse Education Today*, 8, 325–31.

Doherty, G. (1979) The patient in pain: handling the feelings, *Canadian Nurse*, 75(2), 31.

Edwards, W. T. (1990) Optimizing opioid treatment of postoperative pain. *Journal of Pain and Symptom Management*, 5 Feb (1 Supp), S24–36.

Finer (1991) Personal communication, 1991.

Frampton, V. M. (1982) Pain control with the aid of transcutaneous nerve stimulation, *Physiotherapy*, **68**, 77–81.

Francis, I. W. (1987) The Physiology of Pain, in *Nursing the Physically Ill Adult* (eds J. R. P. Boore, R. Champion and M. C. Ferguson), Churchill Livingstone, Edinburgh.

Fagerhaugh, S. Y. and Strauss, A. (1977) *Politics of Pain Management: Staff–Patient Interaction*, Addison-Wesley Publishing Co. Inc., Menlo Park, California.

Hackett, T. P. (1971) Pain and prejudice: Why do we doubt that the patient is in pain? *Medical Times*, **99**(2), 130–41.

Hayward, J. (1975) Information, a prescription against pain. *R.C.N. Research Series.*

Hayward, J. (1979) Pain: psychological and social aspects, *Nursing*, 1, 21–7.

Heimler, E. (1976) *The Storm,* The Menard Press, London.

International Association for the Study of Pain. Subcommittee on education.

Jacox, A. (1977) *Pain: A Source Book for Nurses and Other Health Professionals,* Little, Brown & Co., Boston, Massachusetts.

Kaufman, M. A. and Brown, D. E. (1961) Pain wears many faces, *American Journal of Nursing*, 61, 48–51.

Kleinman, A. (1988) *The Illness Narratives,* Basic Books, New York.

Latham, J. (1990) *Pain Control,* Austen Cornish Ltd with The Lisa Sainsbury Foundation.

Lipton, S. (1979) 'Acupuncture', in *The Control of Chronic Pain* (ed. S. Lipton), Edward Arnold, London.

McCaffery, M. (1980) Understanding your patient's pain, *Nursing*, 80, 26–31.

McCaffery, M. (1983) *Nursing the Patient in Pain,* Lippincott Nursing Series, Harper & Row, London.

McGrath, P. J. and Unruh, A. M. (1987) *Pain in Children and Adolescents,* Elsevier, Amsterdam.

Melzack, R. and Wall, P. D. (1982) *The Challenge of Pain,* Penguin Books, Harmondsworth, Middlesex.

Melzack, R. (1988) The tragedy of needless pain: a call for social action, in *Proc. 5th World Congress on Pain* (eds R. Dubner, G. F. Gebhart and M. R. Bond), Elsevier, Amsterdam, pp. 1–11.

Milton, J. (1972) *Paradise Lost* (ed. J. Broadbent), Cambridge University Press.

Pilowsky, I. and Bond, M. (1969) Pain and its management in malignant disease, *Psychosomatic Medicine*, 31, 400–4.

Seers, K. (1989) Patients' perception of acute pain, in *Directions in Nursing Research* (eds J. Barnett-Wilson and S. Robinson), pp. 107–16. Scutari Press, London.

Sofaer, B. (1983) Pain relief: the core of nursing practice. *Nursing Times*, 79(47), 38–42 and 79(48), 35.

Sofaer, B. (1984) *The Effect of Focused Education for Nursing Teams on Post-operative Pain of Patients.* Unpublished PhD thesis, University of Edinburgh.

Sternbach, R. A. (1968) *Pain: A Psychophysiological Analysis,* Academic Press, New York.

Storlie, F. (1978) Pointers for assessing pain, *Nursing* 78 (May), 37–9.

Taylor, A. G., Skelton, J. and Butcher, J. (1983) Duration of pain, condition and physical pathology: determinants of nurses' assessments of patients in pain. *Nursing Research*, 33, 4–8.

Twycross, R. G. and Lack, S. A. (1983) *Symptom Control for Advanced Cancer: Pain Relief,* Pitman, London.

Wade, J., Price, D. D., Hamer, R. M., Schwartz, S. M. and Hart, R. P. (1990) An emotional component analysis of chronic pain. *Pain*, 40, 303–10.

Walker, J. M., Akinsanya, J. A., Davis, B. D. and Marcer, D. (1989) The nursing management of pain in the community: a theoretical framework. *Journal of Advanced Nursing*, 14, 240–7.

Walker, J. M., Akinsanya, J. A., Davis, B. D. and Marcer, D. (1990) The nursing management of elderly patients with pain in the community: study and recommendations. *Journal of Advanced Nursing*, 15, 1154–61.

Weis, O. F., Sriwatanakul, K., Alloza, J. L., Weintraub, M. and Lasagna, L. (1983) Attitudes of patients, housestaff and nurses towards postoperative analgesic care, *Anesthesia and Analgesia*, **62**(1), 70–4.
Weisenberg, M. (1977) Pain and pain control, *Psychological Bulletin*, **84**(5), 1005–44.

Further reading

Bond, M. R. (1984) *Pain: Its Nature, Analysis and Treatment*, 2nd edn, Churchill Livingstone, Edinburgh.
Fagerhaugh, S. Y. and Strauss, A. (1977) *Politics of Pain Management*, Addison-Wesley Publishing Co. Inc.
Jacox, A. (1977) *Pain: A Source Book for Nurses and Other Health Professionals*, Little, Brown & Co., Boston, Massachusetts.
McCaffery, M. (1983) *Nursing the Patient in Pain*, Harper & Row.
Melzack, R. and Wall, P. D. (1982) *The Challenge of Pain*, Penguin Books Ltd., Middlesex.
Saunders, C. and Baines, M. (1983) *The Management of Terminal Disease*, Oxford Medicine Publications.
Twycross, R. G. and Lack, S. A. (1983) *Symptom Control in Far Advanced Cancer: Pain Relief*, Pitman Books Ltd.

Index

Page numbers in italics refer to figures, and those in bold type to definitions in the glossary